Psychiatry Review for Canadian Doctors

Psychiatry Review for Canadian Doctors

Key preparation for your certification exams

EDITED BY K. SHIVAKUMAR, MD, MRCPSYCH (UK), FRCPC, MPH

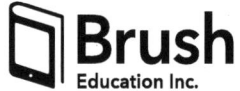

Copyright © 2014 Kuppuswami Shivakumar

22 23 24 25 5 4 3 2

Excerpts from this publication may be reproduced under licence from Access Copyright, or with the express written permission of Brush Education Inc., or under licence from a collective management organization in your territory. All rights are otherwise reserved, and no part of this publication may be reproduced, stored in a retrieval system, or transmitted in any form or by any means, electronic, mechanical, photocopying, digital copying, scanning, recording or otherwise, except as specifically authorized.

Brush Education Inc.
www.brusheducation.ca
contact@brusheducation.ca

Cover design: Dean Pickup; Cover images: Brain icon modified from ID 28509384 © Esignn, Dreamstime.com; Doctor icon from iconsdb.com
Interior design: Carol Dragich, Dragich Design

Printed and manufactured in Canada

Library and Archives Canada Cataloguing in Publication
Psychiatry review for Canadian doctors : key preparation for your certification exams / edited by K. Shivakumar, MD, MRCPsych (UK), FRCPC, MPH.

Includes bibliographical references and index.
Issued in print and electronic formats.
ISBN 978-1-55059-526-0 (pbk.).—ISBN 978-1-55059-452-2 (epub).—
ISBN 978-1-55059-527-7 (pdf).—ISBN 978-1-55059-528-4 (mobi)

1. Psychiatry—Canada—Examinations, questions, etc.   2. Psychiatrists—Certification—Canada.   3. Royal College of Physicians and Surgeons of Canada—Examinations.
I. Shivakumar, K. (Kuppuswami), 1965–, editor

RC440.9.P79 2014   616.890076   C2014-906862-X
                                                             C2014-906863-8

We acknowledge the financial support of the Government of Canada through the Canada Book Fund for our publishing activities.

 Canadian Heritage   Patrimoine canadien

Contents

Preface vii

How to use this book ix

Multiple-choice exam 1 1
Answers: multiple-choice exam 1 13

Multiple-choice exam 2 44
Answers: multiple-choice exam 2 56

Multiple-choice exam 3 87
Answers: multiple-choice exam 3 99

Multiple-choice exam 4 131
Answers: multiple-choice exam 4 142

Case scenarios (OSCE questions) 175

Contributors 253

Index 255

Preface

This book is primarily for psychiatry residents preparing for the certification exams—written and oral—of the Royal College of Physicians and Surgeons of Canada. It is also useful preparation for a variety of other exams, including the psychiatry-resident-in-training examination; and the certification exams in the US, the UK, Australia, and New Zealand.

In addition, the book offers a psychiatry focus for students in other mental health professions and for medical students.

This book is not intended as a textbook. Nor is it purely an examination aid. It offers goal-directed study that engages the format of the Canadian exams and targets key information needed to pass the exam. I believe success in certification exams comes from a structured, disciplined, and consistent approach. This approach is unique to this book in Canada. It is an approach that builds knowledge, skills, and confidence.

I would like to acknowledge with gratitude the contribution of all my colleagues, without whose commitment and enthusiasm this book would not have materialized. All the contributors are experienced psychiatrists with several years of clinical practice. Our primary aim is to provide some practice with taking an exam and to improve candidates' self-confidence. We have drawn on our own clinical experience and on standard psychiatric textbooks to create the questions. We have cited all the materials used in preparing this book, and, in clinical cases, we have not made any reference to any real person, particularly to any of our patients in the past or present.

Thanks to Dr. Katherine Aitchison, who has been a great mentor for me throughout my psychiatric career; the staff of the Health Sciences North library in Sudbury for their tireless work in retrieving several articles; and editor Lynn Zwicky for meticulously reviewing the manuscript and keeping me on track and on schedule with all my tasks. Finally, I would like to acknowledge my summer intern Dominic Cerilli for his excellent literature search skills, and my wife Dr. Ranga Shivakumar for her continuous support and encouragement to complete this book.

It is our hope that this book will help you prepare for your exam and lead you to a successful outcome.

—KS

Disclaimer

The publisher, authors, contributors, and editors bring substantial expertise to this reference and have made their best efforts to ensure that it is useful, accurate, safe, and reliable.

Nonetheless, practitioners must always rely on their own experience, knowledge and judgment when consulting any of the information contained in this reference or employing it in patient care. When using any of this information, they should remain conscious of their responsibility for their own safety and the safety of others, and for the best interests of those in their care.

To the fullest extent of the law, neither the publishers, the authors, the contributors nor the editors assume any liability for injury or damage to persons or property from any use of information or ideas contained in this reference.

How to use this book

The practice exams in this book feature the question formats of the psychiatry certification exam in Canada. This exam has 2 components, set by the Royal College of Physicians and Surgeons of Canada: one written and one oral.

As of spring 2014, the written component comprises only multiple choice questions (no short answer questions).

The oral component is an objective structured clinical exam (OSCE) that approaches questions through case-based scenarios.

Four multiple-choice practice exams

This book features 4 multiple-choice practice exams, each with 50 questions.

The practice exams present all the questions first, without answers. The answers are in sections that follow each exam.

The written component of the qualifying exam itself is a 3-hour exam with around 200 questions. So, you should aim to complete each practice exam in about 45 minutes.

A section of OSCE questions

This book includes 20 OSCE questions, in their own section.

The book presents each question first, followed by answers for each question.

You can approach these questions as short-answer questions: write point-form notes for each and compare your answers to the answers provided.

You can also approach these questions as literal practice for the oral exam, by talking them through with a partner. The partner compares what you say to the answers provided. The advantage of this method is that your partner can also time you. The OSCE component of the qualifying exam is about 4 hours long and divided into "stations" of about 20 minutes each. So, you should spend about 20 minutes completing each question.

Multiple-choice exam 1

1. Which of the following is a risk factor for developing rapid cycling mania?
   a. hyperthyroidism
   b. bipolar II disorder
   c. male gender
   d. depressive episode at onset
   e. shorter duration of illness

2. Which of the following statements is true about buspirone?
   a. It is a partial 5-HT$_{1A}$ antagonist.
   b. It has anticonvulsant properties.
   c. It binds with high affinity to benzodiazepine receptors.
   d. It has extremely high potential for abuse and dependence.
   e. It does not cause sedation in the elderly.

3. Which of the following is not a complication associated with electroconvulsive therapy (ECT)?
   a. arrhythmia
   b. blood pressure changes
   c. changes on electrocardiogram (ECG)
   d. permanent neurological deficits
   e. prolonged seizures

4. Which of the following is true about monoamine oxidase inhibitors (MAOIs)?
   a. The antidepressant activity of MAOIs is directed toward monoamine oxidase B (MAO_B) inhibition.
   b. Monoamine oxidase A (MAO_A) specifically binds to serotonin.
   c. MAO_B specifically binds to norepinephrine.
   d. Dopamine is deaminated more by MAO_A than MAO_B.
   e. Serum monitoring of MAOIs is useful because drug levels correlate with effectiveness.

5. Which of the following statements is true about γ-aminobutyric acid (GABA) receptors?
   a. They are the predominant excitatory receptors in the central nervous system (CNS).
   b. Activation of $GABA_A$ receptors increases the influx of sodium ions into neurons.
   c. Benzodiazepines (BZDs) exert their action by potentiating the activity of the $GABA_B$ receptor complex.
   d. $GABA_B$ receptors are G protein–coupled receptors.
   e. $GABA_C$ receptors are direct-coupled with sodium ion channels.

6. Which of the following statements is true about medications used to treat opioid addiction?
   a. Methadone is a partial agonist.
   b. Buprenorphine is a full agonist.
   c. Naloxone is an opiate agonist.
   d. In contrast to naloxone, naltrexone has a long duration of action.
   e. Naltrexone is contraindicated in renal failure.

7. Which of the following is not a temperamental variable as defined by Alexander Thomas?
   a. activity level
   b. distractibility
   c. low adaptability
   d. intensity of reaction
   e. regularity

8. Which of the following is a feature of normal sleep?
   a. normal respiration
   b. decreased cerebral blood flow
   c. absent tendon reflexes

d. decreased gastric motility
e. preponderance of rapid eye movement (REM) sleep

9. Which of the following is consistent with frontal lobe syndrome?
   a. perseveration
   b. dysphasia
   c. alexia
   d. astereoagnosia
   e. receptive aphasia

10. Which of the following is not true about psychological factors affecting other medical conditions?
    a. A medical condition other than a mental disorder should be present.
    b. There is a clear association between psychological factors affecting other medical conditions and other mental disorders.
    c. The impact of the psychological factors affecting the medical condition can occur at any time during a patient's life.
    d. Cultural factors may influence the presenting features.
    e. Illness anxiety disorder should be excluded in the differential diagnosis.

11. Which of the following descriptions of statistical terminology is correct?
    a. Type I error: This error results from rejecting the null hypothesis when it is in fact false.
    b. Type II error: This error is more serious than a type I error.
    c. P value: Small P values suggest that a null hypothesis is unlikely to be true.
    d. Power: The power of a hypothesis test is the probability of not committing a type I error.
    e. Chi-square test: This test allows comparison of several groups of observations, all of which are independent but possibly with a different mean for each group.

12. Which of the following is a recognized test of frontal lobe function?
    a. Thematic Apperception Test
    b. Rorschach Inkblot Test
    c. Wisconsin Card-Sorting Test
    d. Millon Clinical Multiaxial Inventory
    e. Sentence Completion Test

13. Which of the following is a clinical feature of Prader-Willi syndrome?
    a. hypertonia
    b. hyperphagia
    c. ataxia
    d. spasticity
    e. deleted chromosome of maternal origin

14. Which of the following statements is not true about childhood bipolar disorder?
    a. As in adults, childhood bipolar I disorder requires the existence of a manic or mixed episode.
    b. Childhood bipolar II disorder is characterized by 1 or more major depressive episodes accompanied by at least 1 hypomanic episode.
    c. A hypomanic episode in childhood requires hospital admission.
    d. Children with bipolar disorder may be less responsive to treatment than adults.
    e. Children with bipolar disorder may have a prolonged early course.

15. Which of the following genetic traits have not been associated with conduct disorder?
    a. inattention
    b. somatization
    c. hyperactivity
    d. novelty seeking
    e. aggressiveness

16. Which of the following statements is true about tic disorders?
    a. Tics do not diminish during sleep.
    b. The onset of tics is typically before 8 years of age.
    c. In chronic motor tic disorder, the onset is before 18 years of age.
    d. In Tourette syndrome, the initial symptoms most frequently appear around the time of puberty.
    e. The neuroanatomical substrate of Tourette syndrome is the pituitary gland.

17. Which of the following is not a side effect of psychostimulants?
    a. psychosis
    b. growth delay
    c. decreased appetite
    d. weight loss
    e. sedation

18. Kübler-Ross described 5 stages of reaction in a person facing death. Which of the following is not one of those stages?
    a. anger
    b. reaction formation
    c. bargaining
    d. depression
    e. acceptance

19. Which of the following is not considered a mature defence mechanism?
    a. suppression
    b. humour
    c. altruism
    d. rationalization
    e. sublimation

20. You are seeing a patient in the emergency room. He is drowsy, not responding to pain, and unable to recall any details of his admission. On further examination, his speech is slurred, and he has significant difficulty holding his attention. What is the most likely diagnosis?
    a. opioid withdrawal
    b. LSD intoxication
    c. opioid intoxication
    d. amphetamine withdrawal
    e. phencyclidine intoxication

21. Which of the following statements is true about case control studies?
    a. Case control studies are useful for studying rare exposures.
    b. Relative risk is calculated in case control studies.
    c. It is quick and cheap to conduct a case control study.
    d. Subjects for case control studies are selected according to their exposure.
    e. Nonresponse is a common source of bias in case control studies.

22. Which of the following is an example of retrograde memory loss in an elderly person?
    a. route-finding difficulties
    b. increasing reliance on lists
    c. forgetting recent personal information
    d. losing items around the home
    e. repetitive questioning

23. Which of the following is characteristic of normal pressure hydrocephalus (NPH)?
    a. tremor
    b. bulbar signs
    c. dystonia
    d. fluctuating cognitive impairment
    e. subcortical dementia

24. Which of the following is a core feature of dementia with Lewy bodies (DLB)?
    a. repeated falls
    b. depression
    c. unexplained loss of consciousness
    d. rapid eye movement (REM) sleep behaviour disorder
    e. systematized delusions

25. Which of the following is true about binge-eating disorder?
    a. In binge-eating disorder, compensatory behaviour such as purging and exercise is absent.
    b. Binge-eating episodes occur at least 1 time per month for 6 months.
    c. Self-evaluation is influenced by body shape and image.
    d. It does not occur in normal weight individuals.
    e. It has lower rates of remission than bulimia nervosa.

26. Which of the following is not true about intellectual disability?
    a. It is dependent on IQ scores.
    b. Deficits in adaptive functions such as reading can occur.
    c. Onset of intellectual and adaptive deficits occurs during the developmental period.
    d. The prevalence for severe intellectual disability is approximately 6 in 1000.
    e. Males are more likely than females to be diagnosed with severe forms of intellectual disability.

27. Withdrawal syndrome may occur when selective serotonin reuptake inhibitors (SSRIs) are abruptly stopped, rapidly metabolized, or taken inconsistently. Which of the following is not a withdrawal symptom of SSRIs?
    a. flulike symptoms (myalgia, fatigue)
    b. sleep disturbance (vivid dreams, insomnia)
    c. gastrointestinal problems (nausea, vomiting)

d. sensory disturbances (parenthesis)
e. dry mouth and akathisia

28. In the treatment of disruptive behaviour disorder and aggression among children and adolescents, which of the following psychotropic medications is not used?
    a. olanzapine
    b. aripiprazole
    c. risperidone
    d. methylphenidate
    e. β-blockers

29. Which of the following is not a common reason for treatment failure among adolescents with treatment-resistant depression?
    a. misdiagnosis
    b. inadequate drug dosage or duration of medication trial
    c. noncompliance with treatment
    d. poor therapeutic alliance with physician
    e. presence of bipolar disorder

30. Which of the following factors is a limitation of MAOI combination therapy?
    a. side effects
    b. cost
    c. elimination half-life
    d. skin rashes
    e. protein-binding ability

31. Which of the following is not one of Yalom's curative factors?
    a. universality
    b. denial
    c. altruism
    d. catharsis
    e. imparting information

32. Which of the following statements is not true regarding first-rank symptoms in schizophrenia?
    a. audible thoughts
    b. made impulses
    c. made feelings
    d. restricted affect
    e. thought broadcast

33. Which of the following factors increases suicidal ideation in panic disorder?
   a. old age
   b. late onset of illness
   c. high socioeconomic status
   d. perceived loss of social support
   e. presence of mood disorder

34. Which of the following statements is true about acute dystonic reaction?
   a. Females are at high risk.
   b. It is related to dopamine-receptor blockade.
   c. A feeling of inner restlessness is a common symptom.
   d. Tongue and jaw involvement is much more likely than neck spasm.
   e. History of head injury is a risk factor.

35. Which of the following is a feature of cannabis intoxication?
   a. increased appetite
   b. sweating
   c. incoordination
   d. tremors
   e. blurring of vision

36. Which of the following hematological side effects is associated with carbamazepine?
   a. microcytic anemia
   b. leukocytosis
   c. aplastic anemia
   d. absolute neutrophilia
   e. erythrocytosis

37. Which of the following is not seen in Wernicke encephalopathy?
   a. clear consciousness
   b. ocular palsies
   c. nystagmus
   d. acute degenerative changes in mammillary bodies
   e. staggering gait

38. Which of the following side effects of antidepressants is less common in elderly patients than in younger patients?
   a. postural hypotension
   b. gastric bleeding
   c. inappropriate antidiuretic hormone secretion
   d. increased rates of suicidal behaviour
   e. delirium

39. You are seeing a patient who is suspected of having some prodromal symptoms of psychosis. Which of the following is true about attenuated psychosis syndrome?
   a. For a diagnosis, symptoms must have been present at least daily for the past month.
   b. Psychotic symptoms are more prominent.
   c. The presence of negative symptoms is associated with increased risk of transition to psychosis.
   d. There is a slight female preponderance for attenuated psychosis syndrome.
   e. The majority of individuals with attenuated psychosis syndrome will improve over the time.

40. A 35-year old woman has been treated for recurrent episodes of depression. She has had poor response to treatment and is unable to continue her job. In this patient, which of the following will not cause chronicity of her depression?
   a. personality disorders
   b. comorbid substance abuse
   c. good insight
   d. negative life events
   e. poor compliance with treatment

41. According to evidence from recent studies, which antidepressant is best tolerated and most effective in the elderly population?
   a. venlafaxine
   b. mirtazapine
   c. sertraline
   d. fluoxetine
   e. bupropion

42. Trauma-focused cognitive behavioural therapy (TF-CBT) is recommended for children and adolescents with posttraumatic stress disorder (PTSD). Which of the following is not a component of TF-CBT?
    a. psychoeducation
    b. affirmation
    c. affective modulation skills
    d. trauma narrative
    e. parenting skills

43. Which of the following statements is true about the role of glutamate in obsessive-compulsive disorder (OCD)?
    a. There is evidence to suggest that abnormally low levels of glutamate may contribute to OCD.
    b. Glutamate is an inhibitory neurotransmitter in the brain.
    c. Caudate glutamate is reduced in OCD patients.
    d. Patients with OCD have reduced cerebrospinal fluid glutamate levels.
    e. Memantine modulation of glutamatergic neurotransmission can be used in treating OCD symptoms.

44. Compared to nightmares, which of the following statements about sleep terrors is not true?
    a. Sleep terrors occur during non-REM stage 4 sleep.
    b. Sleep terrors occur during the last third of the night.
    c. Individuals with sleep terrors have no recollection of the event in the morning.
    d. Sleep terrors are effectively treated with sleep hygiene.
    e. Sleep terrors are associated with high arousal thresholds.

45. Which of the following statements is true about augmentation strategies for treatment-resistant depression (TRD)?
    a. Studies have shown that thyroxine (T_4) is superior to L-triiodothyronine (T_3).
    b. Pindolol 5-HT_{1A} agonist has been shown to accelerate response to SSRIs in most double-blinded studies.
    c. Most recent studies have shown a relatively high response rate for lithium augmentation.

d. Augmentation of omega-3 fatty acid to citalopram is a useful strategy for TRD.
e. Double-blinded studies have shown augmenting with inositol in TRD has a good response.

46. Which of the following statements is true about amnesia due to diencephalic and hippocampal lesions?
    a. Perception is impaired.
    b. Immediate memory span is well preserved.
    c. Recent memory is intact.
    d. Performance on test of digit span is usually abnormal.
    e. Procedural memory is not preserved.

47. Which of the following is not a cognitive error?
    a. overgeneralization
    b. personalization
    c. magnification
    d. identification
    e. catastrophic thinking

48. Which of the following medical conditions is not a cause of obsession and compulsion?
    a. post–closed head injury
    b. hyperthyroidism
    c. Huntington disease
    d. Sydenham chorea
    e. anoxia

49. Which of the following conditions is a physiologic effect of cannabis intoxication?
    a. increased libido
    b. hypertension
    c. diarrhea
    d. decreased appetite
    e. bradycardia

50. A 16-year-old girl, diagnosed with complex partial seizure disorder, has been maintained on carbamazepine with adequate seizure control. She developed depressive symptoms and was started on fluoxetine. She then developed diplopia, ataxia, and nausea. On physical examination, she has blood pressure changes and sinus tachycardia. What explains her current presentation?
   a. encephalitis
   b. recurrence of seizure disorder
   c. cytochrome P450 enzyme interaction
   d. migraine
   e. meningitis

ANSWERS: MULTIPLE-CHOICE EXAM 1

1. **Which of the following is a risk factor for developing rapid cycling mania?**
   a. hyperthyroidism
   b. bipolar II disorder
   c. male gender
   d. depressive episode at onset
   e. shorter duration of illness

Answer: b

Dunner and Fieve coined the term *rapid cycling* in 1974. *DSM-5* uses it as a specifier of the longitudinal course of bipolar I or II disorders.

Rapid cycling is defined as 4 mood episodes within 12 months that meet the criteria for a manic, hypomanic, or major depressive episode. Episodes are demarcated by partial or full remission for at least 2 months, or by a switch to an episode of opposite polarity.

Risk factors for rapid cycling include:
- female gender
- bipolar II subtype
- longer duration of illness
- family history of mood disorders
- clinical or subclinical hypothyroidism
- poor response to lithium
- use of antidepressants

READINGS AND REFERENCES

American Psychiatric Association. *Diagnostic and Statistical Manual of Mental Disorders.* 5th ed. Washington, DC: American Psychiatric Publishing; 2013:150–151.

Kupka RW, Luckenbaugh DA, Post RM, et al. Rapid and non-rapid cycling bipolar disorder: a meta-analysis of clinical studies. *J Clin Psychiatry.* 2003;64(12):1483–1494. Medline:14728111

2. **Which of the following statements is true about buspirone?**
   a. It is a partial 5-HT_{1A} antagonist.
   b. It has anticonvulsant properties.
   c. It binds with high affinity to benzodiazepine receptors.
   d. It has extremely high potential for abuse and dependence.
   e. It does not cause sedation in the elderly.

Answer: e

Buspirone hydrochloride is an anxiolytic. It acts as:
- a partial agonist at postsynaptic serotonin (5-HT_{1A}) receptors
- a full agonist at presynaptic 5-HT_{1A} autoreceptors
- a weak antagonist at 5-HT_{2C} receptors

It does not bind to the γ-aminobutyric acid (GABA) benzodiazepine receptor complex; has low potential for abuse; and is generally well tolerated by medically ill elderly patients.

Major side effects of buspirone include headache, nausea, dizziness, and tension. Rare side effects include tachycardia, palpitations, chest pain, drowsiness, confusion, and seizures.

Buspirone does not cause sedation and cognitive impairment in the elderly.

READINGS AND REFERENCES

Sadock BJ, Sadock VA, Ruiz P. *Kaplan and Sadock's Comprehensive Textbook of Psychiatry*. 9th ed. Philadelphia: Lippincott Williams & Wilkins; 2009.

Schatzberg AF, Cole JO, DeBattista C. *Manual of Clinical Psychopharmacology*. 6th ed. Arlington, VA: American Psychiatric Publishing; 2007.

Virani AS, Bezchlibnyk-Butler KZ, Jeffries JJ, Procyshyn RM, eds. *Clinical Handbook of Psychotropic Drugs*. 18th ed. Cambridge, MA: Hogrefe Publishing; 2009:170–173.

3. **Which of the following is not a complication associated with electroconvulsive therapy (ECT)?**
   a. arrhythmia
   b. blood pressure changes
   c. changes on electrocardiogram (ECG)
   d. permanent neurological deficits
   e. prolonged seizures

Answer: d

Some common cardiovascular changes following ECT include: sinus tachycardia; increased blood pressure (more common during unilateral than bilateral); and ST changes on ECG for up to 24 hours. ECT can produce transient neurological deficits. Prolonged seizure, which can occur during the delivery of ECT, is a major complication and should be treated immediately.

READINGS AND REFERENCES

Cristancho MA, Alici Y, Augoustides JG, O'Reardon JP. Uncommon but serious complications associated with electroconvulsive therapy: recognition and management for the clinician. *Curr Psychiatry Rep*. 2008;10(6):474–480. Medline:18980730

4. Which of the following is true about monoamine oxidase inhibitors (MAOIs)?
   a. The antidepressant activity of MAOIs is directed toward monoamine oxidase B (MAO_B) inhibition.
   b. Monoamine oxidase A (MAO_A) specifically binds to serotonin.
   c. MAO_B specifically binds to norepinephrine.
   d. Dopamine is deaminated more by MAO_A than MAO_B.
   e. Serum monitoring of MAOIs is useful because drug levels correlate with effectiveness.

Answer: b

MAOIs differ from each other in enzyme activity. There are 2 subtypes of MAO enzymes: MAO_A and MAO_B. MAO_A inhibitors are considered to have antidepressant activity. The subtypes differ in receptor binding: MAO_A binds more specifically to serotonin and norepinephrine; MAO_B binds specifically with phenylethylamine. Dopamine is equally deaminated by both MAO_A and MAO_B. Serum monitoring of MAOIs is not clinically indicated and drug levels do not correlate with effectiveness.

READINGS AND REFERENCES

Kosinski EC, Rothschild AJ. Forgotten treatment of depression. *Current Psychiatry.* 2012;11(12):21–26.

Rothschild AJ, ed. *The Evidence-Based Guide to Antidepressant Medications.* Arlington, VA: American Psychiatric Publishing; 2012:15–20.

Sadock BJ, Sadock VA. *Kaplan and Sadock's Synopsis of Psychiatry: Behavioral Sciences/Clinical Psychiatry.* 10th ed. Philadelphia: Wolters Kluwer/Lippincott Williams & Wilkins; 2007:1067.

5. Which of the following statements is true about γ-aminobutyric acid (GABA) receptors?
   a. They are the predominant excitatory receptors in the central nervous system (CNS).
   b. Activation of $GABA_A$ receptors increases the influx of sodium ions into neurons.
   c. Benzodiazepines (BZDs) exert their action by potentiating the activity of the $GABA_B$ receptor complex.
   d. $GABA_B$ receptors are G protein–coupled receptors.
   e. $GABA_C$ receptors are direct-coupled with sodium ion channels.

Answer: d

GABA is the major inhibitory neurotransmitter in the CNS. BZDs exert their action by potentiating the activity of $GABA_A$ receptors. They bind to a specific receptor on the $GABA_A$ receptor complex, which facilitates the binding of GABA to its specific receptor site. BZD binding increases the frequency of opening of the chloride channel complexed with the GABA$_A$ receptor. GABA$_B$ receptors increase potassium levels via G protein coupling, whereas GABA$_C$ receptors are direct-coupled receptors with ligand-gated chloride ion channels.

READINGS AND REFERENCES

Puri BK, Hall AD. *Revision Notes in Psychiatry*. 2nd ed. London: Arnold; 2004:229.

Sadock BJ, Sadock VA. *Kaplan and Sadock's Synopsis of Psychiatry: Behavioral Sciences/Clinical Psychiatry*. 10th ed. Philadelphia: Wolters Kluwer/Lippincott Williams & Wilkins; 2007:109.

Wang WW. *Comprehensive Psychiatry Review*. Cambridge: Cambridge University Press; 2010:13.

6. Which of the following statements is true about medications used to treat opioid addiction?
   a. Methadone is a partial agonist.
   b. Buprenorphine is a full agonist.
   c. Naloxone is an opiate agonist.
   d. In contrast to naloxone, naltrexone has a long duration of action.
   e. Naltrexone is contraindicated in renal failure.

Answer: d

For opioid-addiction treatment, opioid agonists and antagonists are commonly used. It is important to differentiate the agents based on their pharmacological activity:

- methadone: full opiate agonist
- buprenorphine: partial opiate agonist
- naloxone: opiate antagonist
- naltrexone: opiate antagonist

Naltrexone can cause dose-related hepatic toxicity: serum aminotransferase levels should be monitored monthly for the first 6 months of naltrexone therapy.

READINGS AND REFERENCES

O'Brien C, Kampman KM. Antagonists of opioids. In: Galanter M, Kleber HD, eds. *The American Psychiatric Publishing Textbook of Substance Abuse Treatment*. 4th ed. Arlington, VA: American Psychiatric Publishing; 2008:325–328.

Sadock BJ, Sadock VA. *Kaplan and Sadock's Synopsis of Psychiatry: Behavioral Sciences/Clinical Psychiatry*. 10th ed. Philadelphia: Wolters Kluwer/Lippincott Williams & Wilkins; 2007:1075.

Virani AS, Bezchlibnyk-Butler KZ, Jeffries JJ, Procyshyn RM, eds. *Clinical Handbook of Psychotropic Drugs*. 18th ed. Cambridge, MA: Hogrefe Publishing; 2009:284–290.

7. **Which of the following is not a temperamental variable as defined by Alexander Thomas?**
   a. activity level
   b. distractibility
   c. low adaptability
   d. intensity of reaction
   e. regularity

Answer: c

Low adaptability is not a temperamental variable as defined by Alexander Thomas and Stella Chess. The New York Longitudinal Study by Thomas and Chess defined 9 temperamental variables:
- activity level
- persistence
- distractibility
- initial reaction
- adaptability
- mood
- intensity of reaction
- sensitivity or sensory threshold
- regularity or rhythmicity

READINGS AND REFERENCES
Chess S, Thomas A, Birch HG. Behavior problems revisited: findings of an anterospective study. *J Am Acad Child Psychiatry*. 1967;6(2):321–331. Medline:6042022
Chrzanowski DT, Gold J. Childhood and adolescent development. In: Ferrando SJ, ed. *Psychiatry In-Review*. 3rd ed. New York: Educational Testing and Assessment Systems (ETAS); 2008:2.

8. **Which of the following is a feature of normal sleep?**
   a. normal respiration
   b. decreased cerebral blood flow
   c. absent tendon reflexes
   d. decreased gastric motility
   e. preponderance of rapid eye movement (REM) sleep

Answer: c

The following are features of normal sleep:
- absent tendon reflexes
- increased blood pressure, gastric motility, and cerebral blood flow
- irregular respiration
- penile erection

- slight tachycardia
- vivid and bizarre dreams

READINGS AND REFERENCES
Buckley P, Prewette D, Bird J, Harrison G. *Examination Notes in Psychiatry*. 4th ed. London: Hodder Arnold; 2005:186.

9. **Which of the following is consistent with frontal lobe syndrome?**
   a. perseveration
   b. dysphasia
   c. alexia
   d. astereoagnosia
   e. receptive aphasia

Answer: a

Frontal lobe syndrome can present with:
- personality changes (common): disinhibition, reduced social and ethical control, facetious humour, sexual indiscretions, poor judgement
- perseveration of actions
- difficulty with programming and planning behaviour

Parietal lobe lesions usually present with:
- cortical sensory loss
- asterognosis
- disorders of body schema: sensory inattention, constructional apraxia, dressing apraxia, topographical agnosia, hemiasomatognosia

Gerstmann syndrome refers to disorders involving the posterior dominant parietal lobe.

READINGS AND REFERENCES
Buckley P, Prewette D, Bird J, Harrison G. *Examination Notes in Psychiatry*. 4th ed. London: Hodder Arnold; 2005:151–153.

10. **Which of the following is not true about psychological factors affecting other medical conditions?**
    a. A medical condition other than a mental disorder should be present.
    b. There is a clear association between psychological factors affecting other medical conditions and other mental disorders.
    c. The impact of the psychological factors affecting the medical condition can occur at any time during a patient's life.
    d. Cultural factors may influence the presenting features.
    e. Illness anxiety disorder should be excluded in the differential diagnosis.

Answer: b

Psychological factors affecting other medical conditions constitute a new entity under somatic symptom and related disorders in *DSM-5*.

As summarized from *DSM-5*, the criteria for this entity include:
- presence of a medical symptom or condition other than a mental disorder
- adverse effect of psychological or behavioural factors on the medical condition in 1 of the following ways:
  - by affecting the course of the condition (close temporal association between psychological factors and onset or exacerbation of condition, or delayed recovery from condition)
  - by interfering with treatment of the condition
  - by generating additional health risks
  - by influencing the underlying psychophysiology
- psychological and behavioural factors not explained by any other mental disorders, such as major depression, posttraumatic stress disorder (PTSD), etc.

In *DSM-5*, somatic symptom and related disorders include:
- somatic symptom disorder
- illness anxiety disorder
- conversion disorder (functional neurological symptom disorder)
- factitious disorder
- other specified somatic symptom and related disorder
- unspecified somatic symptom and related disorder

READINGS AND REFERENCES
American Psychiatric Association. *Diagnostic and Statistical Manual of Mental Disorders.* 5th ed. Washington, DC: American Psychiatric Publishing; 2013:309–327.

11. Which of the following descriptions of statistical terminology is correct?
   a. Type I error: This error results from rejecting the null hypothesis when it is in fact false.
   b. Type II error: This error is more serious than a type I error.
   c. P value: Small P values suggest that a null hypothesis is unlikely to be true.
   d. Power: The power of a hypothesis test is the probability of not committing a type I error.
   e. Chi-square test: This test allows comparison of several groups of observations, all of which are independent but possibly with a different mean for each group.

Answer: c

P value is the probability of erroneously rejecting the null hypothesis.
A type I error is the rejection of a null hypothesis when it is in fact true.
A type II error is the acceptance of a null hypothesis when it is in fact false.
The power of a study is equal to the probability of not making a type II error.

The chi-square test is a nonparametrical test that compares categorical data of the expected frequencies with observed frequencies.

READINGS AND REFERENCES
Lawrie SM, MacIntosh AM, Rao S. *Critical Appraisal for Psychiatrists*. Edinburgh: Elsevier Churchill Livingstone; 2000.

12. Which of the following is a recognized test of frontal lobe function?
    a. Thematic Apperception Test
    b. Rorschach Inkblot Test
    c. Wisconsin Card-Sorting Test
    d. Millon Clinical Multiaxial Inventory
    e. Sentence Completion Test

Answer: c

Many clinicians use the following 2 tests to measure frontal lobe "executive" functioning: the Wisconsin Card-Sorting Test (WCST) and the Trail Making Test, Part B.

The other tests are objective and projective measures of personality in adults.

READINGS AND REFERENCES
Sadock BJ, Sadock VA. *Kaplan and Sadock's Synopsis of Psychiatry: Behavioral Sciences/ Clinical Psychiatry*. 10th ed. Philadelphia: Wolters Kluwer/Lippincott Williams & Wilkins; 2007:181–182.
Stuss DT, Alexander MP. The anatomical basis of affective behavior, emotion and self-awareness: a specific role of the right frontal lobe. In: Hatano G, Okada N, Tanabe H, eds. *Affective Minds: Proceedings of the 13th Toyota Conference*. Amsterdam: Elsevier; 2000:13–25.
Stuss DT, Bisschop SM, Alexander MP, et al. The Trail Making Test: a study in focal lesion patients. *Psychological Assessment*. 2001;13(2):230–239. Medline:11433797

13. Which of the following is a clinical feature of Prader-Willi syndrome?
    a. hypertonia
    b. hyperphagia
    c. ataxia
    d. spasticity
    e. deleted chromosome of maternal origin

Answer: b

The following are features of Prader-Willi syndrome:
- prevalence: 1 in 40 000 live-born infants
- genetic etiology:
  - 70% of cases: deletion in the long arm of chromosome 15 (del 15q11q13), which is always of paternal origin
  - 29% of cases: maternal uniparental disomy (MUPD)
  - 1%: imprinting error
- characterized by:
  - hypotonia
  - obesity (diabetes or heart failure may result)
  - developmental and behavioural problems (including mental retardation)
  - hyperphagia
  - hypogonadism in males
  - dysmorphic features (narrow forehead; down-slanting palpebral fissures; small hands and feet)
  - curvature of the spine or scoliosis (increased prevalence)
  - psychiatric and behavioural disorders (e.g., affective symptoms, psychotic states, anxiety, sleep abnormalities, frequent temper tantrums, self-injury)

READINGS AND REFERENCES
Clarke DM, Shoumitro D. Syndromes causing intellectual disability. In: Gelder MG, Andreasen MD, López-Ibor JJ Jr, Geddes R, eds. *New Oxford Textbook of Psychiatry*. Vol 2. 2nd ed. Oxford: Oxford University Press; 2012:1884.

14. Which of the following statements is not true about childhood bipolar disorder?
   a. As in adults, childhood bipolar I disorder requires the existence of a manic or mixed episode.
   b. Childhood bipolar II disorder is characterized by 1 or more major depressive episodes accompanied by at least 1 hypomanic episode.
   c. A hypomanic episode in childhood requires hospital admission.
   d. Children with bipolar disorder may be less responsive to treatment than adults.
   e. Children with bipolar disorder may have a prolonged early course.

Answer: c

Hypomania in children or in adults does not require hospitalization, and does not significantly impair social or other important functioning. No evidence suggests that children with bipolar disorder are less responsive to treatment than adults; however, youth are highly responsive to second-generation antipsychotics and especially sensitive to their metabolic side effects.

READINGS AND REFERENCES

American Psychiatric Association. *Diagnostic and Statistical Manual of Mental Disorders.* 5th ed. Washington, DC: American Psychiatric Publishing; 2013:123–139.

McGlashan TH. Adolescent versus adult onset of mania. *Am J Psychiatry.* 1988;145(2):221–223. Medline:3124634

Strober M, Schmidt-Lackner S, Freeman R, et al. Recovery and relapse in adolescents with bipolar affective illness: a five-year naturalistic, prospective follow-up. *J Am Acad Child Adolesc Psychiatry.* 1995;34(6):724–731.

Weller EB, Kloos AL, Weller RA. Mood disorders. In: Dulcan M, Wiener J, eds. *Essentials of Child and Adolescent Psychiatry.* Arlington, VA: American Psychiatric Publishing; 2006:253–310.

15. Which of the following genetic traits have not been associated with conduct disorder?

   a. inattention

   b. somatization

   c. hyperactivity

   d. novelty seeking

   e. aggressiveness

Answer: b

Genetic vulnerability to conduct disorder is not yet fully understood. However, several traits are believed to contribute to conduct disorder, including inattention, hyperactivity, aggressiveness, and novelty seeking.

Children diagnosed with conduct disorder often have mothers with antisocial personality, somatization, or problems with alcohol abuse.

READINGS AND REFERENCES

Hendren RL, Mullen DJ. Conduct disorder and oppositional defiant disorder. In: Dulcan M, Wiener J, eds. *Essentials of Child and Adolescent Psychiatry.* Arlington, VA: American Psychiatric Publishing; 2006:357–385.

16. Which of the following statements is true about tic disorders?

   a. Tics do not diminish during sleep.

   b. The onset of tics is typically before 8 years of age.

   c. In chronic motor tic disorder, the onset is before 18 years of age.

   d. In Tourette syndrome, the initial symptoms most frequently appear around the time of puberty.

   e. The neuroanatomical substrate of Tourette syndrome is the pituitary gland.

Answer: c

The following characteristics define tics:

- sudden involuntary, rapid, recurrent, nonrhythmic movements or vocalizations
- diminishment (usually) during sleep or activities that need concentration
- onset: typically between the ages 4 and 6 years
- peak severity: between ages 10 and 12 years (severity declines during adolescence)

According to *DSM-5*, tic disorders include:

- Tourette disorder
- persistent (chronic) motor or vocal tic disorder
- provisional tic disorder
- unspecified tic disorder
- other specified tic disorder

Persistent (chronic) motor or vocal tic disorder involves:

- presence of single or multiple motor or vocal tics, but not both motor and vocal
- onset: before 18 years of age

The basal ganglia and their connections are the most likely neuroanatomical substrate of Tourette disorder.

READINGS AND REFERENCES

American Psychiatric Association. *Diagnostic and Statistical Manual of Mental Disorders.* 5th ed. Washington, DC: American Psychiatric Publishing; 2013:81.

Leckman JF, Riddle MA. Tourette's syndrome. In: Dulcan M, Wiener J, eds. *Essentials of Child and Adolescent Psychiatry.* Arlington, VA: American Psychiatric Publishing; 2006:575.

Leckman JF, Riddle MA. Tourette's syndrome: when habit-forming systems form habits of their own? *Neuron.* 2000;28(2):349–354. Medline:11144345

17. Which of the following is not a side effect of psychostimulants?

   a. psychosis
   b. growth delay
   c. decreased appetite
   d. weight loss
   e. sedation

Answer: e

Psychostimulants such as amphetamine and methylphenidate are mainly used for treating attention deficit hyperactivity disorder (ADHD), narcolepsy, and treatment-resistant depression. In the treatment of ADHD, all psychostimulants have been found equally effective in reducing symptoms.

All of the answers listed in this question, except sedation, are known side effects of psychostimulants.

READINGS AND REFERENCES
Virani AS, Bezchlibnyk-Butler KZ, Jeffries JJ, Procyshyn RM, eds. *Clinical Handbook of Psychotropic Drugs*. 18th ed. Cambridge, MA: Hogrefe Publishing; 2009:216–223.

18. Kübler-Ross described 5 stages of reaction in a person facing death. Which of the following is not one of those stages?

a. anger
b. reaction formation
c. bargaining
d. depression
e. acceptance

Answer: b

The 5 stages of death and dying—reactions to impending death—described by psychiatrist Elizabeth Kübler-Ross are:
- shock and denial
- anger
- bargaining
- depression
- acceptance

READINGS AND REFERENCES
Kübler-Ross E. *On Death and Dying*. New York: Scribner; 1969.
Sadock BJ, Sadock VA. *Kaplan and Sadock's Synopsis of Psychiatry: Behavioral Sciences/ Clinical Psychiatry*. 10th ed. Philadelphia: Wolters Kluwer/Lippincott Williams & Wilkins; 2007:62–63.

19. Which of the following is not considered a mature defence mechanism?

a. suppression
b. humour
c. altruism
d. rationalization
e. sublimation

Answer: d

The following are mature defence mechanisms:
- suppression: consciously avoiding painful thoughts or feelings
- humour: treating unpleasant experiences as funny or ironic
- altruism: responding to painful thoughts or feelings by attending to the needs of others
- anticipation: focusing on future needs
- compensation: developing abilities that make up for deficits
- sublimation: converting unacceptable impulses into socially acceptable behaviours

READINGS AND REFERENCES
Sussman C, Khatkhate G, Tavares A, et al. Psychotherapy. In: Kupfer DJ, Horner MS, Brent DA, et al, eds. *Oxford American Handbook of Psychiatry*. Oxford: Oxford University Press; 2008:997–998.

20. You are seeing a patient in the emergency room. He is drowsy, not responding to pain, and unable to recall any details of his admission. On further examination, his speech is slurred, and he has significant difficulty holding his attention. What is the most likely diagnosis?
    a. opioid withdrawal
    b. LSD intoxication
    c. opioid intoxication
    d. amphetamine withdrawal
    e. phencyclidine intoxication

Answer: c

In the presence of other indicators of recent opioid use, the following strongly suggest opioid intoxication:
- altered mood
- psychomotor retardation
- drowsiness
- slurred speech
- impaired memory and attention with hallucinatory experiences (in the absence of delirium)

Note that *DSM-5* lists the following specifier: opioid intoxication with perceptual disturbances.

READINGS AND REFERENCES
American Psychiatric Association. *Diagnostic and Statistical Manual of Mental Disorders*. 5th ed. Washington, DC; American Psychiatric Publishing: 2013:546.

21. Which of the following statements is true about case control studies?
a. Case control studies are useful for studying rare exposures.
b. Relative risk is calculated in case control studies.
c. It is quick and cheap to conduct a case control study.
d. Subjects for case control studies are selected according to their exposure.
e. Nonresponse is a common source of bias in case control studies.

Answer: c

Features of case control studies include:
- Subjects are selected according to their caseness (by contrast, in cohort studies, subjects are selected according to their exposure).
- Subjects retrospectively recall exposure.
- Selection and information bias is elevated in case control studies.
- It is quick and relatively cheap to do a case control study.
- Case control studies are useful for rare and single outcomes with multiple exposures.
- The odds ratio is calculated in case control studies (by contrast, relative risk is calculated in cohort studies).

READINGS AND REFERENCES
Prince M. Epidemiology. In: Jacoby R, Oppenheimer C, Dening T, Thomas A, eds. *Oxford Textbook of Old Age Psychiatry*. Oxford: Oxford University Press; 2008:59.

22. Which of the following is an example of retrograde memory loss in an elderly person?
a. route-finding difficulties
b. increasing reliance on lists
c. forgetting recent personal information
d. losing items around the home
e. repetitive questioning

Answer: a

Symptoms suggestive of anterograde memory loss include:
- increasing reliance on lists
- forgetting recent personal information
- losing items around the home
- repetitive questioning
- inability to follow or remember story plots (e.g., television shows, movies) or current affairs

Retrograde memory loss may involve:
- losing memories of past events
- getting physically lost

READINGS AND REFERENCES
Kipps CM, Hodges JR. Clinical cognitive assessment. In: Jacoby R, Oppenheimer C, Dening T, Thomas A, eds. *Oxford Textbook of Old Age Psychiatry*. Oxford: Oxford University Press; 2008;156–157.

23. Which of the following is characteristic of normal pressure hydrocephalus (NPH)?
a. tremor
b. bulbar signs
c. dystonia
d. fluctuating cognitive impairment
e. subcortical dementia

Answer: d

NPH has a triad of clinical characteristics: incontinence, gait disturbance, and fluctuating cognitive impairment. Computed tomography (CT) findings include: large lateral ventricles, a small fourth ventricle, periventricular hypodensities, a small superior interhemispheric fissure, and small sulci.

Magnetic resonance imaging (MRI) shows the typical "fluid void sign" (this sign is characteristic but nonspecific—it also occurs in 30% of the healthy elderly).

Wilson disease is characterized by tremor, dystonia, bulbar signs (dysphagia, dysarthria), and subcortical dementia.

READINGS AND REFERENCES
Hentschel F, Förstl H. Neuroimaging and neurophysiology in the elderly. In: Jacoby R, Oppenheimer C, Dening T, Thomas A, eds. *Oxford Textbook of Old Age Psychiatry*. Oxford: Oxford University Press; 2008:188.

24. Which of the following is a core feature of dementia with Lewy bodies (DLB)?
a. repeated falls
b. depression
c. unexplained loss of consciousness
d. rapid eye movement (REM) sleep behaviour disorder
e. systematized delusions

Answer: d

The following are core diagnostic features of DLB:
- visual hallucinations
- fluctuation of cognition
- spontaneous parkinsonism
- REM sleep behaviour disorder
- neuroleptic sensitivity
- repeated falls and syncope
- transient, unexplained loss of consciousness
- severe autonomic dysfunction (orthostatic hypotension)
- hallucinations in other modalities
- systematized delusions
- depression

READINGS AND REFERENCES

Hentschel F, Förstl H. Neuroimaging and neurophysiology in the elderly. In: Jacoby R, Oppenheimer C, Dening T, Thomas A, eds. *Oxford Textbook of Old Age Psychiatry.* Oxford: Oxford University Press; 2008:185.

McKeith IG, Dickson DW, Lowe J, et al. Diagnosis and management of dementia with Lewy bodies: third report of the DLB Consortium. *Neurology.* 2005;65(12):1863–1872. Medline:16237129

McKeith IG, Galasko D, Kosaka K, et al. Consensus guidelines for the clinical and pathological diagnosis of dementia with Lewy bodies (DLB): report of the Consortium on DLB International Workshop. *Neurology.* 1996;47(5):1113–1124. Medline:8909416

25. Which of the following is true about binge-eating disorder?
   a. In binge-eating disorder, compensatory behaviour such as purging and exercise is absent.
   b. Binge-eating episodes occur at least 1 time per month for 6 months.
   c. Self-evaluation is influenced by body shape and image.
   d. It does not occur in normal weight individuals.
   e. It has lower rates of remission than bulimia nervosa.

Answer: a

According to *DSM-5*, 3 or more of the following are associated with binge-eating disorder (Criterion B):
- eating much more rapidly than normal
- eating until uncomfortably full

- eating large amounts when not hungry
- eating alone because of embarassment
- feeling disgusted with oneself

The binge eating occurs, on average, 1 time per week for 3 months (Criterion D).

In bulimia nervosa, self-evaluation is unduly influenced by body shape and weight.

Binge-eating disorder occurs in normal weight, overweight, and obese individuals.

In both natural-course and treatment-outcome studies, remission rates are higher for binge-eating disorder than for bulimia nervosa or anorexia nervosa.

READINGS AND REFERENCES
American Psychiatric Association. *Diagnostic and Statistical Manual of Mental Disorders.* 5th ed. Washington, DC: American Psychiatric Publishing; 2013:338–353.

26. **Which of the following is not true about intellectual disability?**
    a. It is dependent on intelligence quotient (IQ) scores.
    b. Deficits in adaptive functions such as reading can occur.
    c. Onset of intellectual and adaptive deficits occurs during the developmental period.
    d. The prevalence for severe intellectual disability is approximately 6 in 1000.
    e. Males are more likely than females to be diagnosed with severe forms of intellectual disability.

Answer: a

All other statements are true.

READINGS AND REFERENCES
American Psychiatric Association. *Diagnostic and Statistical Manual of Mental Disorders.* 5th ed. Washington, DC: American Psychiatric Publishing; 2013:33–41.

27. **Withdrawal syndrome may occur when selective serotonin reuptake inhibitors (SSRIs) are abruptly stopped, rapidly metabolized, or taken inconsistently. Which of the following is not a withdrawal symptom of SSRIs?**
    a. flulike symptoms (myalgia, fatigue)
    b. sleep disturbance (vivid dreams, insomnia)
    c. gastrointestinal problems (nausea, vomiting)
    d. sensory disturbances (parenthesis)
    e. dry mouth and akathisia

Answer: e

In addition to flulike symptoms, sleep disturbance, gastrointestinal problems, and sensory disturbances, SSRI withdrawal can also produce disequilibrium problems. Escitalopram has fewer withdrawal symptoms than paroxetine. Fluoxetine has fewer withdrawal symptoms than drugs with shorter half-lives such as citalopram, fluvoxamine, paroxetine, and venlafaxine.

READINGS AND REFERENCES
Schatzberg AF, Haddad P, Kaplan EM, et al. Serotonin reuptake inhibitor discontinuation syndrome: a hypothetical definition. Discontinuation consensus panel. *J Clin Psychiatry*. 1997;58(suppl 7):5–10. Medline:9219487

28. In the treatment of disruptive behaviour disorder and aggression among children and adolescents, which of the following psychotropic medications is not used?
    a. olanzapine
    b. aripiprazole
    c. risperidone
    d. methylphenidate
    e. β-blockers

Answer: e

Risperidone (effect size: 0.9) is the most studied medication to treat aggression among children and adolescents, followed by aripiprazole (effect size: 0.87).

Risperidone and aripiprazole have become first-line medications, replacing typical antipsychotic medications. Typical antipsychotics increase the risk of extrapyramidal symptoms (EPS) and tardive dyskinesia.

READINGS AND REFERENCES
Zaraa SG, Cunningham NR, Pappadopulos E, Jensen PS. Disruptive behavior disorders and aggression. In: McVoy M, Findling, RL, eds. *Clinical Manual of Child and Adolescent Psychopharmacology*. 2nd ed. Arlington, VA: American Psychiatric Publishing; 2012:97–135.

29. Which of the following is not a common reason for treatment failure among adolescents with treatment-resistant depression?
    a. misdiagnosis
    b. inadequate drug dosage or duration of medication trial
    c. noncompliance with treatment
    d. poor therapeutic alliance with physician
    e. presence of bipolar disorder

Answer: d

The initial step in managing patients with treatment-resistant depression is to establish nonresponse. The next step is to determine the reasons for nonresponse, which may include the presence of comorbid psychiatric or medical illnesses—e.g., dysthymia, anxiety, attention-deficit/hyperactivity disorder (ADHD), substance use, personality disorder, hypothyroidism. Other factors include severe depression, suicidality, exposure to negative events such as abuse, and hopelessness.

READINGS AND REFERENCES
Birmaher B. Major depressive disorder. In: McVoy M, Findling, RL, eds. *Clinical Manual of Child and Adolescent Psychopharmacology.* 2nd ed. Arlington, VA: American Psychiatric Publishing; 2012:191–217.

30. Which of the following factors is a limitation on MAOI combination therapy?
    a. side effects
    b. cost
    c. elimination half-life
    d. skin rashes
    e. protein-binding ability

Answer: a

The side effects of MAOIs are the major limitation on MAOI use in regular clinical practice. Side effects are thought to arise from the interaction of MAOIs with foods high in tyramine and other monoamines.

MAOIs are relatively cheap compared to other antidepressants. They generally have a shorter plasma elimination half-life than other antidepressants (note, however, that comparisons of elimination half-life and protein binding are not relevant in the case of irreversible MAOIs, because of their irreversible effects on monoamine oxidase). MAOIs are all rapidly absorbed.

READINGS AND REFERENCES
Bhagwagar Z, Heninger GR. Antidepressants. In: Gelder MG, Andreasen MD, López-Ibor JJ Jr, Geddes R, eds. *New Oxford Textbook of Psychiatry.* Vol 2. 2nd ed. Oxford: Oxford University Press; 2012:1185–1190.

31. Which of the following is not one of Yalom's curative factors?
    a. universality
    b. denial
    c. altruism
    d. catharsis
    e. imparting information

Answer: b

On the basis of research done on the phases of small groups, Yalom tabulated the curative factors in a group's life, which include:
- initiation of hope
- universality
- imparting information
- altruism
- corrective recapitulation of primary family group
- development of socializing techniques
- imitative behaviour
- interpersonal learning
- group cohesiveness
- catharsis
- existential factors

READINGS AND REFERENCES

Schlapobersky J, Pines M. Group methods in adult psychiatry. In: Gelder MG, Andreasen MD, López-Ibor JJ Jr, Geddes R, eds. *New Oxford Textbook of Psychiatry*. Vol 2. 2nd ed. Oxford: Oxford University Press; 2012:1355–1356.

Yalom ID. *The Theory and Practice of Group Psychotherapy*. 4th ed. New York: Basic Books; 1995.

32. Which of the following statements is not true regarding first-rank symptoms in schizophrenia?
   a. audible thoughts
   b. made impulses
   c. made feelings
   d. restricted affect
   e. thought broadcast

Answer: d

According to Schneiderian criteria, the following are first-rank symptoms of schizophrenia: audible thoughts, somatic passivity, thought insertion, thought withdrawal, thought broadcast, made feelings, made impulses, made volition, voices arguing, voices commenting, and delusional perception. Restricted affect is part of the negative symptoms.

READINGS AND REFERENCES

Sadock BJ, Sadock VA. *Kaplan and Sadock's Synopsis of Psychiatry: Behavioral Sciences/ Clinical Psychiatry*. 10th ed. Philadelphia: Wolters Kluwer/Lippincott Williams & Wilkins; 2007:468.

33. **Which of the following factors increases suicidal ideation in panic disorder?**
    a. old age
    b. late onset of illness
    c. high socioeconomic status
    d. perceived loss of social support
    e. presence of mood disorder

Answer: d

According to a study by Huang, Yen, and Lung, factors that increase suicidal ideation in panic disorder include:

- younger age
- early onset of illness
- socioeconomic status (low)
- alcohol use (current)
- severity of panic symptoms (increasing)
- availability of social support (perceived as decreasing)
- adverse side effects of medication (perceived as increasing)

READINGS AND REFERENCES

Antar LM, Hollander E. Anxiety disorders. In: Simon RI, Hales RE, eds. *The American Psychiatric Publishing Textbook of Suicide Assessment and Management*. 2nd ed. Arlington, VA: American Psychiatric Publishing; 2012:124.

Huang MF, Yen CF, Lung FW. Moderators and mediators among panic, agoraphobia symptoms, and suicidal ideation in patients with panic disorder. *Comprehensive Psychiatry*. 2010;51(3):243–249. Medline:20399333

34. **Which of the following statements is true about acute dystonic reaction?**
    a. Females are at high risk.
    b. It is related to dopamine-receptor blockade.
    c. A feeling of inner restlessness is a common symptom.
    d. Tongue and jaw involvement is much more likely than neck spasm.
    e. History of head injury is a risk factor.

Answer: b

Medication-induced movement disorders are common and important to consider in a differential diagnosis.

Acute dystonic reaction produces painful muscular spasms and twisted abnormal postures. Symptoms can begin immediately, or can be delayed for hours or days. Most cases occur within the first 5 days.

Acute dystonic reaction mostly follows the introduction of antipsychotics. Those at a higher risk include: males, people with a personal or family history of dystonia, and younger people. Other risk factors include: liver failure, clinically severe schizophrenia, and the use of high-potency antipsychotics.

Akathisia causes a subjective feeling of inner restlessness or tension with attentional dysfunction, anxiety, discomfort, depression, paranoia, and impulsivity.

READINGS AND REFERENCES
Strassnig M, Rock JE, Patterson KR, Stowell KR. Therapeutic issues. In: Kupfer DJ, Horner MS, Brent DA, et al, eds. *Oxford American Handbook of Psychiatry*. Oxford: Oxford University Press; 2008:1058–1064.

35. Which of the following is a clinical feature of cannabis intoxication?
    a. increased appetite
    b. sweating
    c. incoordination
    d. tremors
    e. blurring of vision

Answer: a

In an acute clinical situation, it is important to differentiate withdrawal and intoxication. It is also common to see more than 1 substance involved at a time.

Cannabis intoxication usually occurs within 2 hours of cannabis use. The most common symptoms are conjunctival injection, increased appetite, dry mouth, and tachycardia.

Cannabis withdrawal develops within 1 week after discontinuing heavy cannabis use. Common symptoms include irritability, anger, aggression, nervousness, sleep problems, weight loss (or loss of appetite), restlessness, and depressed mood. Physical symptoms can include abdominal pain, shakiness, tremor, sweating, fever, chills, or headache—and again these should be differentiated from opioid withdrawal symptoms.

Pupillary dilatation, tachycardia, sweating, palpitations, blurring of vision, tremors, and incoordination are features of hallucinogen intoxication.

READINGS AND REFERENCES
American Psychiatric Association. *Diagnostic and Statistical Manual of Mental Disorders*. 5th ed. Washington, DC: American Psychiatric Publishing; 2013:516–529.

36. Which of the following hematological side effects is associated with carbamazepine?
    a. microcytic anemia
    b. leukocytosis

c. aplastic anemia
d. absolute neutrophilia
e. erythrocytosis

Answer: c

Several hematological side effects are associated with carbamazepine therapy, including agranulocytosis, aplastic anemia, transitory leukopenia, persistent leukopenia, thrombocytopenia, purpura, and anemia.

READINGS AND REFERENCES
Pellock JM. Carbamazepine side effects in children and adults. *Epilepsia*. 1987; 28 (supplement 3): S64–S70. Medline:2961558
Virani AS, Bezchlibnyk-Butler KZ, Jeffries JJ, Procyshyn RM, eds. *Clinical Handbook of Psychotropic Drugs*. 18th ed. Cambridge, MA: Hogrefe Publishing; 2009:200.

37. **Which of the following is not seen in Wernicke encephalopathy?**
    a. clear consciousness
    b. ocular palsies
    c. nystagmus
    d. acute degenerative changes in mammillary bodies
    e. staggering gait

Answer: a

Thiamine deficiency causes Wernicke encephalopathy, which involves acute degenerative changes in the thalamus, hypothalamus, and mammillary bodies. Clinical signs include confusion, clouding of consciousness, ocular palsies, nystagmus, staggering gait, and peripheral neuropathy. Ataxia and ocular symptoms typically resolve quickly with thiamine treatment.

READINGS AND REFERENCES
Buckley P, Prewette D, Bird J, Harrison G. *Examination Notes in Psychiatry*. 4th ed. London: Hodder Arnold; 2005:114–115.

38. **Which of the following side effects of antidepressants is less common in elderly patients than in younger patients?**
    a. postural hypotension
    b. gastric bleeding
    c. inappropriate antidiuretic hormone secretion
    d. increased rates of suicidal behaviour
    e. delirium

Answer: d

All of the side effects listed in this question are commonly associated with antidepressant therapy in elderly patients. However, studies of antidepressant therapy have reported higher rates of self-harm and suicidal behaviour in pediatric patients and adults younger than 25.

READINGS AND REFERENCES
Baldwin RC. *Depression in Late Life*. Oxford Psychiatry Library. Oxford: Oxford University Press; 2010.
Virani AS, Bezchlibnyk-Butler KZ, Jeffries JJ, Procyshyn RM, eds. *Clinical Handbook of Psychotropic Drugs*. 18th ed. Cambridge, MA: Hogrefe Publishing; 2009:2–16.

39. **You are seeing a patient who is suspected of having some prodromal symptoms of psychosis. Which of the following is true about attenuated psychosis syndrome?**
    a. For a diagnosis, symptoms must have been present at least daily for the past month.
    b. Psychotic symptoms are more prominent.
    c. The presence of negative symptoms is associated with increased risk of transition to psychosis.
    d. There is a slight female preponderance for attenuated psychosis syndrome.
    e. The majority of individuals with attenuated psychosis syndrome will improve over the time.

Answer: c

DSM-5 describes attenuated psychotic symptoms as similar to psychotic symptoms, but well below the threshold of a psychotic disorder. The psychotic symptoms are transient and less severe. For a diagnosis of attenuated psychosis syndrome, symptoms must be present at least once per week for the past month. Males are slightly more likely than females to suffer from attenuated psychosis syndrome. According to the literature, most individuals will improve over time. Factors that increase the risk of transition to psychosis include negative symptoms, cognitive impairment, and poor functioning.

READINGS AND REFERENCES
American Psychiatric Association. *Diagnostic and Statistical Manual of Mental Disorders*. 5th ed. Washington, DC: American Psychiatric Publishing; 2013:783–786.

40. **A 35-year old woman has been treated for recurrent episodes of depression. She has had poor response to treatment and is unable to continue her job. In this patient, which of the following will not cause chronicity of her depression?**
    a. personality disorders
    b. comorbid substance abuse
    c. good insight

d. negative life events

e. poor compliance with treatment

Answer: c

All the factors listed above will prolong the patient's depression and lead to chronicity except for good insight. Good insight generally improves the prognosis as well as the treatment response.

READINGS AND REFERENCES
Keitner GI, Mansfield AK. Management of treatment-resistant depression. *Psychiatr Clin N Am*. 2012;35(1):249–265. Medline:22370501

41. According to evidence from recent studies, which antidepressant is best tolerated and most effective in the elderly population?

   a. venlafaxine
   b. mirtazapine
   c. sertraline
   d. fluoxetine
   e. bupropion

Answer: c

According to a study by Cipriani et al., sertraline shows slightly superior tolerability and effectiveness for treating depression in the elderly.

READINGS AND REFERENCES
Cipriani A, La Ferla T, Furukawa TA, et al. Sertraline versus other antidepressive agents for depression. *Cochrane Database Syst Rev*. 2010; issue 4;Art No CD006117. doi:10.1002/14651858.CD006117.pub4. Medline:20393946

42. Trauma-focused cognitive behavioural therapy (TF-CBT) is recommended for children and adolescents with PTSD. Which of the following is not a component of TF-CBT?

   a. psychoeducation
   b. affirmation
   c. affective modulation skills
   d. trauma narrative
   e. parenting skills

Answer: b

The components of TF-CBT include (mnemonic: **P-PRACTICE**):

- **p**sychoeducation
- **p**arenting skills
- **r**elaxation skills

- affective modulation skills
- cognitive coping and processing
- trauma narrative
- in vivo mastery of trauma reminders
- conjoint child-parent sessions
- enhancing future safety and development

Affirmation is part of motivation in interviewing.

READINGS AND REFERENCES

Cohen JA, Bukstein O, Walter H, et al. Practice parameters for the assessment and treatment of children and adolescents with posttraumatic stress disorder. *Journal of the American Academy of Child and Adolescent Psychiatry.* 2010;49(4):414–430. Medline:20410735

43. Which of the following statements is true about the role of glutamate in obsessive-compulsive disorder (OCD)?
    a. There is evidence to suggest that abnormally low levels of glutamate may contribute to OCD.
    b. Glutamate is an inhibitory neurotransmitter in the brain.
    c. Caudate glutamate is reduced in OCD patients.
    d. Patients with OCD have reduced cerebrospinal fluid glutamate levels.
    e. Memantine modulation of glutamatergic neurotransmission can be used in treating OCD symptoms.

Answer: e

A single-blinded case control study of memantine in severe OCD by Stewart et al. showed an improvement of OCD symptoms compared to controls. Current clinical pharmacological studies modulating glutamatergic neurotransmission show that memantine, riluzole, and N-acetylcysteine have a role in treating OCD patients. Riluzole has been used as an augmenting agent in treatment-resistant OCD; a study by Coric et al. showed some patients with treatment-resistant OCD reduced their Yale-Brown Obsessive Compulsive Scale (Y-BOCS) scores by more than 35%. Glutamate is the most abundant excitatory neurotransmitter in the brain and the levels are abnormally elevated in OCD. Caudate glutamate is elevated in OCD patients before treatment and decreases after effective treatment.

READINGS AND REFERENCES

Chakrabarty K, Bhattacharyya S, Christopher R, Khanna S. Glutamatergic dysfunction in OCD. *Neuropsychopharmacology.* 2005;30(9):1735–1740. Medline:15841109

Coric V, Taskiran S, Pittenger C, et al. Riluzole augmentation in treatment-resistant obsessive-compulsive disorder: an open-label trial. *Biol Psychiatry.* 2005;58(5):424–428. Medline:15993857

Stewart SE, Jenike EA, Hezel DM, et al. A single-blinded case-control study of memantine in severe obsessive-compulsive disorder. *J Clin Psycho Pharmacol.* 2010;30(1):34–39. Medline:20075645

44. Compared to nightmares, which of the following statements about sleep terrors is not true?

a. Sleep terrors occur during non-REM stage 4 sleep.
b. Sleep terrors occur during the last third of the night.
c. Individuals with sleep terrors have no recollection of the event in the morning.
d. Sleep terrors are effectively treated with sleep hygiene.
e. Sleep terrors are associated with high arousal thresholds.

Answer: b

Sleep terrors occur during the first third of the night when non-REM stage 4 sleep predominates.

Nightmares occur during the REM stage. They are frightening to the individual and they occur in the early morning hours, particularly after 2 a.m. Individuals who experience nightmares recall them the following morning.

READINGS AND REFERENCES
Mindell JA, Owens JA. *A Clinical Guide to Pediatric Sleep Diagnosis and Management of Sleep Problems.* 2nd ed. Philadelphia: Wolters Kluwer/Lippincott Williams & Wilkins; 2010:82.

45. Which of the following statements is true about augmentation strategies for treatment-resistant depression (TRD)?

a. Studies have shown that thyroxine (T_4) is superior to L-triiodothyronine (T_3).
b. Pindolol 5-HT_{1A} agonist has been shown to accelerate response to SSRIs in most double-blinded studies.
c. Most recent studies have shown a relatively high response rate for lithium augmentation.
d. Augmentation of omega-3 fatty acid to citalopram is a useful strategy for TRD.
e. Double-blinded studies have shown augmenting with inositol in TRD has a good response.

Answer: d

Common strategies for TRD include: switching, dose increase, augmentation, and combination.

Augmentation enhances the effect of an antidepressant. In TRD, common augmentation agents include lithium, thyroid, pindolol, atypical antipsychotics, and modafinil. Interest has also recently emerged for the following agents: methylfolate, amantadine, ketamine, scopolamine, riluzole, D-cycloserine, inositol, and S-adenosylmethionine (SAMe).

Thyroid hormone augmentation (25–50 mcg per day) is a useful strategy in treatment-resistant depression. L-triiodothyronine (T_3) has been preferentially used and thought to be superior to thyroxine (T_4).

Pindolol is a β-blocker, and a 5-HT_{1A} antagonist (not an agonist). It has been shown to accelerate response to SSRIs in most double-blinded studies.

Although it is a common strategy to use lithium to augment the effect of an antidepressant, a study by Fava et al. showed—interestingly—no significant relationship between lithium levels and degree of improvement as measured by HAM-D 17 scores.

A double-blinded study by Nemets et al. failed to support the use of inositol (up to 12 g per day) in treatment-resistant depression.

READINGS AND REFERENCES

Aronson R, Offman HJ, Joffe RT, Naylor CD. Triiodothyronine augmentation in the treatment of refractory depression: a meta-analysis. *Arch Gen Psychiatry*. 1996;53(9):842–848. Medline:8792761

Ballesteros J, Callado LF. Effectiveness of pindolol plus serotonin uptake inhibitors in depression: a meta-analysis of early and late outcomes from randomised controlled trials. *Journal of Affective Disorders*. 2004;79(1–3):137. Medline:15023488

Blier P, Bergeron R. The use of pindolol to potentiate antidepressant medication. *J Clin Psychiatry*. 1998;59(suppl 5):16. Medline:9635544

Fava M, Alpert J, Nierenberg A, et al. Double-blind study of high-dose fluoxetine versus lithium or desipramine augmentation of fluoxetine in partial responders and nonresponders to fluoxetine. *J Clin Psychopharmacol*. 2002;22(4):379–387. Medline:12172337

Gertsik L, Poland RE, Bresee C, Rapaport MH. Omega-3 fatty acid augmentation of citalopram treatment for patients with major depressive disorder. *J Clin Psychopharmacol*. 2012;32(1):61–64. Medline:22198441

Joffe RT, Singer W. A comparison of triiodothyronine and thyroxine in the potentiation of tricyclic antidepressants. *Psychiatry Res*. 1990;32(3):241–251. Medline:2201988

Nemets B, Mishory A, Levine J, Belmaker RH. Inositol addition does not improve depression in SSRI treatment failures. *J Neural Transm*. 1999;106(7–8):795–798. Medline:10907738

46. Which of the following statements is true about amnesia due to diencephalic and hippocampal lesions?

a. Perception is impaired.

b. Immediate memory span is well preserved.

c. Recent memory is intact.

d. Performance on test of digit span is usually abnormal.

e. Procedural memory is not preserved.

Answer: b

Lesions in the hypothalamic-diencephalic system or in the hippocampal regions cause similar memory deficits. The following signs may occur with hypothalamic-diencephalic lesions:
- impaired perception
- well-preserved immediate memory span
- perseveration of the immediate memory span (clinically important)
- normal performance on digit span test
- defective recent memory
- well-preserved procedural memory

READINGS AND REFERENCES
Lishman WA. *Organic Psychiatry: The Psychological Consequences of Cerebral Disorders*. 3rd ed. Oxford: Blackwell Science; 1988:29–32.

47. Which of the following is not a cognitive error?
   a. overgeneralization
   b. personalization
   c. magnification
   d. identification
   e. catastrophic thinking

Answer: d

A goal of cognitive behavioural therapy (CBT) is to shape the content of automatic thoughts by identifying "cognitive errors" or distortions. In addition to overgeneralization, personalization, magnification, and catastrophic thinking, some other cognitive errors are all-or-none thinking, selective negative focus, and jumping to conclusions.

READINGS AND REFERENCES
Kay J, Tasman A. *Essentials of Psychiatry*. Chichester, UK: John Wiley & Sons; 2006:873.

48. Which of the following medical conditions is not a cause of obsession and compulsion?
   a. post–closed head injury
   b. hyperthyroidism
   c. Huntington disease
   d. Sydenham chorea
   e. anoxia

Answer: b

Obsession and compulsion occur as part of many psychiatric disorders. They also occur in the context of some general medical conditions and medical treatments, for example post–encephalitic lesions, post–anoxic state, post–closed head injury, treatment with clozapine, Sydenham chorea, and Huntington disease.

READINGS AND REFERENCES
Kay J, Tasman A. *Essentials of Psychiatry*. Chichester, UK: John Wiley & Sons; 2006:401.

49. Which of the following conditions is a physiologic effect of cannabis intoxication?
    a. increased libido
    b. hypertension
    c. diarrhea
    d. decreased appetite
    e. bradycardia

Answer: b

Cannabis intoxication is associated with physical and psychological intoxication.

Tachycardia, hypertension, thirst, increased appetite, constipation, decreased libido, and mydriasis are some of the known physiologic effects of cannabis intoxication.

Euphoria, dysphoria, restlessness, depersonalization, derealization, and paranoid ideas are known psychological effects of cannabis intoxication.

READINGS AND REFERENCES
Kay J, Tasman A. *Essentials of Psychiatry*. Chichester, UK: John Wiley & Sons; 2006:441.

50. A 16-year-old girl, diagnosed with complex partial seizure disorder, has been maintained on carbamazepine with adequate seizure control. She developed depressive symptoms and was started on fluoxetine. She then developed diplopia, ataxia, and nausea. On physical examination, she has blood pressure changes and sinus tachycardia. What explains her current presentation?
    a. encephalitis
    b. recurrence of seizure disorder
    c. cytochrome P450 enzyme interaction
    d. migraine
    e. meningitis

Answer: c

This patient is showing signs of carbamazepine toxicity.

Carbamazepine is metabolized through the cytochrome P450 3A3 and 3A4 enzyme (CYP3A3, CYP3A4) system. Fluoxetine and fluvoxamine increase plasma levels of carbamazepine, so carbamazepine levels should be carefully monitored when starting these antidepressants. Other medications that can increase carbamazepine include: valproic acid, tricyclic antidepressants, macrolide antibiotics, and prednisolone.

READINGS AND REFERENCES

Thomas T, Kuich KW, Findling R. Anticonvulsants. In: McVoy M, Findling R, eds. *Clinical Manual of Child and Adolescent Psychopharmacology*. 2nd ed. Arlington, VA: American Psychiatric Publishing; 2013:235–239.

Multiple-choice exam 2

1. **Which of the following statements is true about alcoholic hallucinosis?**
   a. Alcoholic hallucinations present as auditory hallucinations in the context of an altered sensorium.
   b. Delusions of grandeur form part of alcoholic hallucinations.
   c. Alcoholic hallucinations occur in most patients with severe alcohol withdrawal.
   d. They are a form of schizophrenia.
   e. They are classified as a substance-induced psychotic disorder.

2. **Which of the following statements about acamprosate is true?**
   a. It is structurally similar to N-methyl-D-aspartic acid (NMDA).
   b. Constipation is a side effect of acamprosate.
   c. Dosage adjustment is not required in hepatic disorders.
   d. It has a pharmacokinetic interaction with alcohol.
   e. Sudden discontinuation is associated with withdrawal syndrome and should be avoided.

3. **Which of the following statements is true about pyromania?**
   a. A person who has purposefully set a fire on more than 1 occasion can be diagnosed with pyromania.
   b. It is a dissociative disorder.
   c. Pyromania as a primary diagnosis is very common.
   d. There is a direct relationship between fire setting and mental disorders.
   e. Most arsonists fulfill criteria for psychosis.

4. Which of the following is a contraindication for electroconvulsive therapy (ECT)?
   a. neuroleptic malignant syndrome not responding to medication
   b. severe depression with psychotic features
   c. medical conditions with raised intracranial pressure
   d. intractable epilepsy not responding to anticonvulsants
   e. depression due to dementia

5. Which of the following statements is true about Margaret Mahler's separation/individualism theory?
   a. Margaret Mahler described a 5-stage process of separation-individuation.
   b. The second stage of differentiation starts from 5 to 10 months of age.
   c. During the stage of practicing, infants become more cognizant of their own bodies.
   d. The final stage—the stage of rapprochement—develops between 18 and 24 months of age.
   e. Consolidation and object constancy develop between 24 and 36 months of age.

6. Which of the following is true about ECT?
   a. The mortality rate after ECT treatment is about 1 in 10 000.
   b. The intensity of the shock administered is not related to the extent of cognitive impairment.
   c. Unilateral ECT results in high remission rates.
   d. Seizure thresholds do not change during the treatment course.
   e. Lithium therapy can be safely continued for ECT patients.

7. Which of the following is true about psychiatric disorders and suicide risk?
   a. Suicide rates are significantly elevated with bulimia nervosa.
   b. Suicide risk is increased in patients with major depressive disorder with melancholic features compared to patients with major depressive disorder.
   c. Panic disorder is not associated with an increased risk of suicidal ideation.
   d. Lower intelligence quotient (IQ) influences the risk of suicide in patients with posttraumatic stress disorder (PTSD).
   e. Religious obsessions are not associated with an increased risk of suicide in patients with obsessive-compulsive disorder (OCD).

8. Which of the following is true about electroencephalogram (EEG) findings?
    a. Delta waves can be seen in nonsleeping adults.
    b. Alpha waves are accentuated by eye closure.
    c. Theta waves are always abnormal.
    d. The frequency of alpha waves is greater than beta waves.
    e. Benzodiazepines slow beta waves.

9. Which of the following statements is true about psychiatric rating scales?
    a. The Present State Examination (PSE) covers symptoms in the last 6 to 8 weeks.
    b. The General Health Questionnaire (GHQ) is a clinician-rated instrument.
    c. The Brief Psychiatric Rating Scale (BPRS) produces subscores for affective, psychotic, and negative symptoms.
    d. BPRS is a self-rated scale.
    e. BPRS is a highly reliable standardized test.

10. Which of the following is a "core" diagnostic feature of frontotemporal lobar degeneration (FTD)?
    a. slow onset
    b. early loss of insight
    c. hyperorality
    d. perseverative behaviour
    e. utilization behaviour

11. Which of the following findings is true about dementia with Lewy bodies (DLB)?
    a. It is more prevalent in females.
    b. Lewy bodies are eosinophilic extra cytoplasmic inclusion bodies.
    c. Early loss of language is common.
    d. Extrapyramidal symptoms (EPS) are reported in 25% to 50% of DLB cases.
    e. Patients with DLB generally perform poorly on tests of verbal memory.

12. Which of the following findings is not seen in normal pressure hydrocephalus (NPH)?
    a. ataxia
    b. urinary incontinence

c. irreversible dementia
d. normal cerebrospinal fluid pressure
e. progressive slowing of cognitive function

13. Which of the following statements is true about cortical dementia compared to subcortical dementia?
    a. slowed cognitive processing
    b. prominent psychomotor retardation
    c. gait disturbance
    d. severe depression
    e. significant memory impairment

14. Which of the following rating scales is used in assessing externalizing behaviours?
    a. Child Behavior Checklist (CBCL)
    b. Conners Rating Scale
    c. Mania Rating Scale
    d. Beck Depression Inventory
    e. Children's Depression Rating Scale

15. Which of the following syndromes is not correctly paired with its chromosomal abnormality?
    a. Prader-Willi syndrome: deletion of chromosome 15 of paternal origin
    b. fragile X syndrome: fragile site on the long (q) arm of the X chromosome at Xq27.3
    c. cri du chat syndrome: deletion of chromosome at 5p15.2 of paternal origin
    d. Down syndrome: trisomy 18
    e. Angelman syndrome: deletion within 15q11q13 of maternal origin

16. Which of the following is true of patients who have early onset bipolar disorder?
    a. They have higher rates of psychotic features than those with onset at an older age.
    b. Early onset of symptoms indicates a shorter course of illness.
    c. Children with bipolar disorder are more responsive to treatment than adults.
    d. Grandiose delusions are more common than paranoid delusions.
    e. Euphoria is more common than irritability and unpredictable mood.

17. Mothers of children diagnosed with conduct disorder are more likely to have which of the following conditions?
    a. somatization
    b. criminal behaviour
    c. anxiety disorders
    d. depression
    e. bipolar disorder

18. Which of the following is true about Tourette syndrome?
    a. Both multiple tics and 1 or more vocal tics should be present.
    b. Coprolalia is a common early symptom.
    c. It is more common in girls.
    d. It is usually associated with psychotic symptoms.
    e. Treatment with D_2 receptor antagonists usually completely suppresses the tics.

19. Which of the following author-theory pairings is correct?
    a. Rogers: object relations theory
    b. Klein: transactional analysis
    c. Berne: client centred therapy
    d. Erikson: alternative model of psychosocial development
    e. Winnicot: theories of childhood development, including primitive defence

20. Which of the following is not a characteristic test for frontal lobe function?
    a. Category Fluency Test
    b. Go-No-Go task
    c. Cognitive Estimate Test
    d. reproducing interlocking pentagons
    e. Luria test

21. Which of the following neuroimaging findings does not indicate vascular dementia?
    a. ischemic infarction
    b. subcortical vascular encephalopathy
    c. fornix infarcts
    d. amyloid angiopathy
    e. bilateral thalamic hyperintensity

22. Which of the following statements is true about cholinesterase inhibitors?
    a. Galantamine is an irreversible competitive inhibitor of acetylcholinesterase.
    b. Memantine is effective in mild Alzheimer disease.
    c. The effects of cholinesterase inhibitors on behavioural disturbances are dose dependent.
    d. Donepezil is an irreversible inhibitor of acetylcholinesterase.
    e. Rivastigmine is a pseudo-irreversible inhibitor of acetylcholinesterase.

23. Which of the following is true about sleep changes in elderly patients (older than 65)?
    a. shorter sleep latency
    b. shorter rapid eye movement (REM) latency
    c. increased total sleep time
    d. less stage 1 and 2 sleep
    e. more slow-wave sleep

24. Which of the following is not a characteristic of a positive family history for alcoholism?
    a. family history of depression
    b. conduct disorder during childhood
    c. deficit in executive cognitive functioning
    d. attention-deficit/hyperactivity disorder (ADHD) as a child
    e. low educational achievement

25. A meta-analysis of published and unpublished randomized control trials of antidepressants assessed the number needed to treat (NNT) to achieve benefits from antidepressants. The antidepressants studied were selective serotonin reuptake inhibitors (SSRIs) and serotonin-norepinephrine reuptake inhibitors (SNRIs). What value did the study find for the NNT?
    a. 5%
    b. 10%
    c. 15%
    d. 20%
    e. 25%

26. The US National Institute of Mental Health (NIMH) conducted a study of methylphenidate among 3- to 5-year-olds: the Preschool ADHD Treatment Study (PATS). Which of the following is not a finding of the study?
   a. Methylphenidate is effective in preschoolers with ADHD.
   b. Eleven percent of subjects withdrew from the study because of adverse events.
   c. Methylphenidate resulted in lower rates of emotional adverse events (e.g., irritability and crying episodes) in the study group compared to older children.
   d. The mean optimal dose of methylphenidate was lower than the mean optimal dose for school-age children.
   e. Preschoolers metabolized methylphenidate slower than school-age children.

27. A major US study of therapies for pediatric obsessive-compulsive disorder—the Pediatric OCD Treatment Study (POTS)—evaluated the acute efficacy of sertraline, cognitive behavioural therapy (CBT), combination treatment (CBT and sertraline), and placebo. Which of the following statements is not a conclusion of the study?
   a. Response to CBT, sertraline, and combination treatment was significantly greater than placebo.
   b. Response to combination treatment was superior to CBT or sertraline alone.
   c. The remission rate for combination treatment was lower compared to sertraline, CBT, or placebo.
   d. The remission rate for sertraline was not different from placebo.
   e. The remission rate for CBT was not different from sertraline, but was greater than placebo.

28. Benzodiazepines are used for anxiety disorders. Which of the following statements is not true regarding the mechanism of action of benzodiazepines?
   a. Benzodiazepine receptors appear to be part of the membrane complexes involving chloride channels and γ-aminobutyric (GABA) receptors.
   b. At these sites, benzodiazepines bind to larger protein complexes found on the receptors and facilitate $GABA_B$ transmission, which leads to increased chloride conductance and increased inhibition of the central nervous system (CNS).
   c. Benzodiazepines lower serotonin turnover and activity.

d. Benzodiazepines lower the spontaneous firing of noradrenergic neurons in the locus coeruleus.
e. Benzodiazepines decrease dopaminergic function.

29. Because of the possible cardiac effects of stimulants, physicians need to check the personal and family history of children and adolescents before treating them with stimulants. Which of the following is not relevant in this context?
    a. tetralogy of Fallot
    b. cardiac artery abnormalities
    c. obstructive subaortic stenosis
    d. edema of the lower extremities
    e. previous consultation with a cardiologist

30. Which of the following statements about mood stabilizers is true?
    a. Carbamazepine doses need to be increased when used in combination with valproate.
    b. Valproate doubles lamotrigine levels when used in combination, so dosing should be one-half that of normal.
    c. Carbamazepine is a weak 3A4 inducer.
    d. Inhibition of 3A4 will notably decrease carbamazepine levels.
    e. Carbamazepine increases levels of haloperidol when used in combination.

31. Which of the following statements is true about brief psychotic disorder?
    a. The average age of onset is mid-20s.
    b. Symptoms last at least 1 day but not longer than 1 week.
    c. It is twice as common in females.
    d. Paranoid personality disorder is a risk factor for developing brief psychotic disorder.
    e. The outcome is usually poor due to difficulties in social functioning.

32. Which of the following brain regions is involved in OCD?
    a. amygdala
    b. cerebellum
    c. basal ganglia
    d. hypothalamus
    e. locus coeruleus

33. Which of the following statements about gabapentin is true?
    a. It exerts its effects through direct regulation of benzodiazepine receptors.
    b. It has a benign drug-interaction profile with no active metabolites.
    c. It has significant cytochrome P450 interactions.
    d. It acts as a GABA precursor.
    e. It has excellent protein-binding capacity.

34. Which of the following is true about culture-bound disorders?
    a. Koro is mostly associated with Mexico.
    b. Windigo involves fear of engaging in cannibalism.
    c. Latah is the belief that the penis will retract into the abdomen and cause death.
    d. Amok has a history in Malaysia and is an anxiety-associated condition.
    e. Automatic obedience hypersuggestibility is seen in frigophobia.

35. Which of the following statements is true about speech disturbances associated with schizophrenia?
    a. logoclonia
    b. stuttering
    c. dysarthria
    d. cryptolalia
    e. aphonia

36. Which of the following is true of depressive disorder with melancholic features?
    a. hypersomnia
    b. significant anorexia
    c. leaden paralysis
    d. mood reactivity
    e. affective flattening

37. Which of the following symptoms is suggestive of delirium rather than dementia?
    a. insidious onset
    b. progressive course
    c. fixed delusions
    d. incongruity of mood
    e. labile affect

38. Which of the following is a sign of acute phencyclidine intoxication?
   a. hypotension
   b. bradycardia
   c. pinpoint pupils
   d. nystagmus
   e. respiratory arrest with a pulse

39. Which of the following antidepressants is associated with fewer sexual side effects?
   a. bupropion
   b. paroxetine
   c. venlafaxine
   d. fluoxetine
   e. fluvoxamine

40. A 70-year old man presents with worsening forgetfulness and is unable to keep his appointments. Which of the following would suggest a mild cognitive impairment in this patient?
   a. evidence of significant cortical dysfunction
   b. changes in his activities of daily living
   c. objective memory impairment for his age
   d. evidence suggestive of dementia
   e. changes in mood

41. Which of the following is a protective factor against persistence of violence?
   a. being last-born
   b. coming from a large family
   c. being an active and affective infant
   d. low IQ
   e. exposure to parental conflict

42. Which of the following factors is not associated with poor prognosis in anorexia nervosa?
   a. older age of onset
   b. longer duration of illness
   c. personality problems
   d. good family support
   e. bulimic features

43. Which of the following conditions should not be considered in the differential diagnosis of a patient with body dysmorphic disorder?
    a. major depressive disorder
    b. obsessive-compulsive personality disorder (OCPD)
    c. schizophrenia
    d. social phobia
    e. trichotillomania

44. According to the Social Readjustment Rating Scale, which of the following life changes is considered highly stressful?
    a. death of a spouse
    b. divorce
    c. retirement from work
    d. death of a close family member
    e. detention in jail

45. Which of the following statements about brief focal psychotherapy is true?
    a. Resolution of the Oedipus complex is part of the therapy.
    b. Duration is 12 treatment hours.
    c. Challenging defenses is the primary focus of therapy.
    d. Catharsis is promoted.
    e. Linking the past, the present, and the transference is important.

46. Which of the following statements about neuroleptic malignant syndrome (NMS) is true?
    a. The onset of NMS is rapid.
    b. Hyperkinesia is seen.
    c. NMS progresses rapidly.
    d. Muscle rigidity is commonly seen.
    e. NMS is more common in women.

47. Which of the following symptoms is most commonly seen in patients with PTSD?
    a. anxiety at reminders of the trauma
    b. recurrent nightmares
    c. insomnia
    d. restricted affect
    e. increased use of alcohol

48. Which of the following is true about cardiovascular changes associated with aging?
    a. increase in heart size
    b. increase in flexibility of the collagen matrix
    c. fat destruction in the myocardium
    d. increased left ventricular diastolic filling
    e. reduced peak exercise index and ejection fraction

49. Which of the following statements is true about the use of neuroleptics for OCD?
    a. First-generation neuroleptics are usually helpful.
    b. Second-generation agents such as risperidone can be used as monotherapy.
    c. Neuroleptics may worsen OCD symptoms if used without an SSRI.
    d. Neuroleptics are the primary choice of treatment for OCD.
    e. For ODC patients, neuroleptics act more quickly than SSRIs.

50. Which of the following is a side effect of carbamazepine that commonly diminishes with a temporary reduction in dose?
    a. agranulocytosis
    b. aplastic anemia
    c. lupus erythematous–like syndrome
    d. pulmonary hypersensitivity
    e. headache

ANSWERS: MULTIPLE-CHOICE EXAM 2

1. **Which of the following statements is true about alcoholic hallucinosis?**
   a. Alcoholic hallucinations present as auditory hallucinations in the context of an altered sensorium.
   b. Delusions of grandeur form part of alcoholic hallucinations.
   c. Alcoholic hallucinations occur in most patients with severe alcohol withdrawal.
   d. They are a form of schizophrenia.
   e. They are classified as a substance-induced psychotic disorder.

   Answer: e
   Alcoholic hallucinosis is a rare condition and occurs in 3% to 10% of patients with severe alcohol withdrawal. It can present as auditory, visual, or tactile hallucinations in the presence of a clear sensorium after abrupt cessation of heavy drinking. The hallucinations are fragmentary to start with, but soon become second- or third-person auditory hallucinations. The voices tend to threaten or abuse. *DSM-5* classifies alcoholic hallucinosis as a substance-induced psychotic disorder and not, as has been suggested in the past, a form of schizophrenia.

   The condition lasts about 1 week and clears spontaneously in several months. It usually develops in patients with long-term alcohol abuse or dependence. Treatment usually entails benzodiazepines, improved nutritional status, fluids, and, if the symptoms are severe, high potency antipsychotics. The hallucinations usually respond rapidly to antipsychotic agents. The prognosis is good. Symptoms that last for 6 months generally continue for years.

   READINGS AND REFERENCES
   Glass IB. Alcoholic hallucinosis: a psychiatric enigma—1. The development of an idea. *Br J Addict.* 1989;84(1):29–41. Medline:2644996
   Leamon MH, Wright TM, Myron H. Substance-related disorders. In: Bourgeois JA, Hales RE, Young JS, et al, eds. *The American Psychiatric Publishing Board Review Guide for Psychiatry.* Arlington, VA: American Psychiatric Publishing; 2009:256.
   Mann KF, Kiefer F. Alcohol and psychiatric and physical disorders. In: Gelder MG, Andreasen MD, López-Ibor JJ Jr, Geddes R, eds. *New Oxford Textbook of Psychiatry.* Vol 1. Oxford, UK: Oxford University Press; 2012:443.
   Strahl NR. *Clinical Study Guide for the Oral Boards in Psychiatry.* 2nd edition. Arlington, VA: American Psychiatric Publishing; 2005:284.

2. **Which of the following statements about acamprosate is true?**
   a. It is structurally similar to *N*-methyl-D-aspartic acid (NMDA).
   b. Constipation is a side effect of acamprosate.

c. Dosage adjustment is not required in hepatic disorders.
  d. It has a pharmacokinetic interaction with alcohol.
  e. Sudden discontinuation is associated with withdrawal syndrome and should be avoided.

Answer: c

Acamprosate is structurally similar to γ-aminobutyric acid (GABA) and is thought to decrease the effects of naturally occurring excitatory neurotransmitter glutamate. Sudden alcohol abstinence results in an unopposed excitatory effect of glutamate on the increased number of NMDA receptors. This mechanism appears to play a significant role in the pathophysiology of alcohol withdrawal syndrome and acamprosate is believed to counteract this type of glutamate effect.

No dosage adjustment is required in hepatic disorders because acamprosate is not metabolized by the liver; it is excreted unexchanged in urine. Acamprosate should be avoided in severe renal insufficiency. It is not associated with any withdrawal syndrome. The most common adverse effects are nausea, flatulence and diarrhea, headache, asthenia, and pruritus.

READINGS AND REFERENCES
Sadock BJ, Sadock VA. *Kaplan and Sadock's Synopsis of Psychiatry: Behavioral Sciences/Clinical Psychiatry*. 10th ed. Philadelphia: Wolters Kluwer/Lippincott Williams & Wilkins; 2007:1039–1040.
Virani AS, Bezchlibnyk-Butler KZ, Jeffries JJ, Procyshyn RM, eds. *Clinical Handbook of Psychotropic Drugs*. 18th ed. Toronto: Hogrefe Publishing; 2009:282.

3. Which of the following statements is true about pyromania?
  a. A person who has purposefully set a fire on more than 1 occasion can be diagnosed with pyromania.
  b. It is a dissociative disorder.
  c. Pyromania as a primary diagnosis is very common.
  d. There is a direct relationship between fire setting and mental disorders.
  e. Most arsonists fulfill criteria for psychosis.

Answer: a

Pyromania is defined as a pattern of deliberate fire setting for pleasure or satisfaction, which is derived from the relief of tension experienced before fires are set. A person who has purposefully set a fire on more than 1 occasion can be diagnosed with pyromania.

A person with pyromania exhibits fascination, curiosity, or attraction with regard to the fires they set and the situational context of the fires (e.g., method of setting, purpose, outcome). *DSM-5* classifies pyromania under disruptive impulse-control and conduct disorders (other disorders in this classification include oppositional defiant disorder, intermittent explosive disorder, and kleptomania). Psychosis can occur with fire setting, but there is a high co-occurrence of substance-use disorders, gambling disorder, depressive disorders, and bipolar disorders.

READINGS AND REFERENCES
American Psychiatric Association. *Diagnostic and Statistical Manual of Mental Disorders.* 5th ed. Washington, DC: American Psychiatric Publishing; 2013:476–477.

Eastman N, Adshead G, Fox S, et al. *Forensic Psychiatry.* Oxford Specialist Handbooks in Psychiatry. Oxford: Oxford University Press; 2012:38–39.

4. Which of the following is a contraindication for electroconvulsive therapy (ECT)?
a. neuroleptic malignant syndrome not responding to medication
b. severe depression with psychotic features
c. medical conditions with raised intracranial pressure
d. intractable epilepsy not responding to anticonvulsants
e. depression due to dementia

Answer: c

All major clinical guidelines accept the following conditions as indications for ECT:
- depression
- mania
- schizophrenia
- catatonia
- neuroleptic malignant syndrome
- intractable epilepsy

ECT can improve tremor, rigidity, bradykinesia, and gait in Parkinson disease for periods of several weeks, but is rarely used for this indication. Any conditions associated with raised intracranial pressure are known contraindications to ECT.

READINGS AND REFERENCES
George MS, Nabas ZH, Borckardt JJ, et al. Nonpharmacological somatic treatments. In: Bourgeois JA, Hales RE, Young JS, et al, eds. *The American Psychiatric Publishing Board Review Guide for Psychiatry.* Arlington, VA: American Psychiatric Publishing; 2009:575.

Kennedy R, Mittal D, O'Jile J. Electroconvulsive therapy in movement disorders: an update. *J Neuropsychiatry Clin Neurosci.* 2003;15(4):407–421. Medline:14627767

5. Which of the following statements is true about Margaret Mahler's separation/individualism theory?
   a. Margaret Mahler described a 5-stage process of separation-individuation.
   b. The second stage of differentiation starts from 5 to 10 months of age.
   c. During the stage of practicing, infants become more cognizant of their own bodies.
   d. The final stage—the stage of rapprochement—develops between 18 and 24 months of age.
   e. Consolidation and object constancy develop between 24 and 36 months of age.

Answer: e

Margaret Mahler described the process by which infants and children differentiate themselves from their primary caregivers.

Mahler describes a 4-stage process of separation/individuation that develops during the first 3 years of life:

- stage of differentiation: 5 to 10 months; infants become more cognizant of their own bodies and begin to move away from their mothers physically
- stage of practicing: 10 to 15 months
- stage of rapprochement: 18 to 24 months
- consolidation and object constancy: 24 to 36 months

READINGS AND REFERENCES

Chrzanowski DT, Gold J. Childhood and adolescent development. In: Ferrando SJ, ed. *Psychiatry In-Review*. 3rd ed. New York: Educational Testing and Assessment Systems (ETAS); 2008:2–3.

Mahler MS, Pine F, Bergman A. *The Psychological Birth of the Human Infant: Symbiosis and Individuation*. New York: Basic Books; 1975.

6. Which of the following is true about ECT treatment?
   a. The mortality rate after ECT treatment is about 1 in 10 000.
   b. The intensity of the shock administered is not related to the extent of cognitive impairment.
   c. Unilateral ECT results in high remission rates.
   d. Seizure thresholds do not change during the treatment course.
   e. Lithium therapy can be safely continued for ECT patients.

Answer: a

ECT is generally a safe treatment when performed under general anesthesia. The risk of serious complications is about 1 in 1000, and the risk of death is about 1 in 10 000.

The cognitive effects of ECT remain an issue of concern and controversy. ECT may cause 3 types of memory disturbances: acute confusional state, retrograde amnesia, and anterograde amnesia. The extent of cognitive impairment (primarily retrograde amnesia) is proportional to the intensity of the shock administered.

Changes in seizure threshold occur in less than 20% of patients during the treatment course and seizure thresholds increase during the treatment course. Therefore, seizures should be monitored during treatment.

Lithium combined with ECT can result in confusional states, serotonin syndrome, and prolonged and/or focal seizures. For acute ECT, it is safe to discontinue lithium. For continuation and maintenance ECT, lithium is usually withheld for 24 hours before treatment.

READINGS AND REFERENCES
Petrides G, Fink M, Husain MM, et al. ECT remission rates in psychotic versus nonpsychotic depressed patients: a report from CORE. *J ECT*. 2001;17(4):244–253. Medline:11731725
Sadock BJ, Sadock VA. *Kaplan and Sadock's Comprehensive Textbook of Psychiatry: Behavioral Sciences/Clinical Psychiatry*. 9th ed. Philadelphia: Wolters Kluwer/Lippincott Williams & Wilkins; 2007:3285–3301.

7. **Which of the following is true about psychiatric disorders and suicide risk?**
   a. Suicide rates are significantly elevated with bulimia nervosa.
   b. Suicide risk is increased in patients with major depressive disorder with melancholic features compared to patients with major depressive disorder.
   c. Panic disorder is not associated with an increased risk of suicidal ideation.
   d. Lower IQ influences the risk of suicide in patients with posttraumatic stress disorder (PTSD).
   e. Religious obsessions are not associated with an increased risk of suicide in patients with obsessive-compulsive disorder (OCD).

Answer: b

Suicide risk is increased in patients with major depressive disorder with melancholic features compared to patients with major depressive disorder. A study by Grunebaum et al. compared suicide attempts associated with melancholic versus nonmelancholic major depression; it showed that melancholic patients had more serious suicide attempts, and increased probability and lethality of future attempts.

Suicide rates are not significantly elevated in patients with bulimia nervosa; however, they are high in patients with anorexia nervosa.

In the absence of other comorbidities, panic disorder increases the risk of suicide. In patients with panic disorders, certain clinical factors may act synergistically to increase suicide risk, including:

- younger age
- early onset of illness
- socioeconomic status (low)
- alcohol use (current)
- severity of panic symptoms (increasing)
- availability of social support (perceived as decreasing)
- adverse side effects of medication (perceived as increasing)

Higher IQ and comorbid psychiatric disorders influence the risk of suicide attempts in patients with PTSD.

OCD is associated with increased risk of suicide. Certain obsessions increase the risk of suicide in OCD patients, including religious obsession, sexual obsession, symmetry obsessions, ordering obsessions, repeating compulsions, and reassurance-seeking compulsions.

READINGS AND REFERENCES

Antar LM, Hollander E. Anxiety disorders. In: Simon RI, Hales RE, eds. *The American Psychiatric Publishing Textbook of Suicide Assessment and Management*. 2nd ed. Arlington, VA: American Psychiatric Publishing; 2012:123–141.

Grunebaum MF, Galfalvy HC, Oquendo MA, et al. Melancholia and the probability and lethality of suicide attempts. *Br J Psychiatry*. 2004;184(June):534–535. Medline:15172948

Huang MF, Yen CF, Lung FW. Moderators and mediators among panic, agoraphobia symptoms, and suicidal ideation in patients with panic disorder. *Comprehensive Psychiatry*. 2010;51(3):243–249. Medline:20399333

Kotler M, Iancu I, Efroni R, Amir M. Anger, impulsivity, social support, and suicide risk in patients with posttraumatic stress disorder. *J Nerv Ment Dis*. 2001;189(3):162–167. Medline:11277352

Pompili M, Mancinelli I, Girardi P, et al. Suicide and attempted suicide in anorexia nervosa and bulimia nervosa. *Ann Ist Sup Sanita*. 2003;39(2):275–81. Medline:14587228

8. **Which of the following is true about electroencephalogram (EEG) findings?**
   a. Delta waves can be seen in nonsleeping adults.
   b. Alpha waves are accentuated by eye closure.
   c. Theta waves are always abnormal.

d. The frequency of alpha waves is greater than beta waves.

e. Benzodiazepines slow beta waves.

Answer: b

Electroencephalography records waves in the following ranges:
- amplitude: 5 µV to 150 µV
- frequency: ~1 Hz to > 40 Hz

A normal EEG usually consists of approximately 7 types of waves. The breakdown that follows describes the 4 basic wave forms.

WAVE FORM	RANGE	NOTES
Delta	< 4 Hz	These are invariably abnormal in nonsleeping adults
Theta	4 to 7 Hz	Transient theta waves can be found in 15% of the normal population
Alpha	8 to 13 Hz	These are: • prominent over the occipital region • accentuated by eye closure • attenuated by attention
Beta	≥ 14 Hz	These may be enhanced by anxiety, alcohol, barbiturates, and benzodiazepines

READINGS AND REFERENCES

Buckley P, Prewette D, Bird J, Harrison G. *Examination Notes in Psychiatry*. 4th ed. London: Hodder Arnold; 2005:185.

9. Which of the following statements is true about psychiatric rating scales?

a. The Present State Examination (PSE) covers symptoms in the last 6 to 8 weeks.

b. The General Health Questionnaire (GHQ) is a clinician-rated instrument.

c. The Brief Psychiatric Rating Scale (BPRS) produces subscores for affective, psychotic, and negative symptoms.

d. BPRS is a self-rated scale.

e. BPRS is a highly reliable standardized test.

Answer: c

BPRS measures psychotic symptoms and psychopathology through a 16-item structured interview. Each item is scored on a 7-point scale. It is an observer-rated instrument, so it is less reliable than a standardized test.

GHQ measures current mental health. It was originally a 60-item self-rated instrument; shorter versions are now available. The questionnaire asks respondents whether they have experienced particular symptoms or behaviours recently. It is not suitable for detection of psychosis.

PSE is a semistructured interview that covers symptoms during the previous 4 weeks.

READINGS AND REFERENCES

Goldberg DP. *The Detection of Psychiatric Illness by Questionnaire*. Oxford: Oxford University Press; 1972.

Goldberg DP, Blackwell B. Psychiatric illness in general practice: a detailed study using a new method of case identification. *Br Med J*. May 23, 1970; 2(5707):439–443. Medline:5420206

Overall JE, Gorham DR. The brief psychiatric rating scale. *Psychological Reports*. 1962;10(2):799–812.

Tress KH, Bellenis C, Brownlow JM, et al. The present state examination change rating scale. *Br J Psychiatry*. February 1987:150:201–207. Medline:3651674

10. Which of the following is a "core" diagnostic feature of frontotemporal lobar degeneration (FTD)?

a. slow onset
b. early loss of insight
c. hyperorality
d. perseverative behaviour
e. utilization behaviour

Answer: b

FTD diagnosis is based on international criteria. It is a progressive disorder with insidious onset, affective symptoms, language disorder, frontal executive dysfunction with preserved spatial orientation, and selective frontotemporal atrophy or hypoperfusion/hypometabolism.

Clinically, FTD is diagnosed via core and supportive diagnostic features. The core diagnostic features of FTD are:

- insidious onset and gradual progression
- early decline in social interpersonal conduct
- early impairment in regulation of personal conduct
- early emotional blunting
- early loss of insight

Supportive diagnostic features include:

- behavioural disorder
- decline in personal hygiene
- mental rigidity

- distractibility
- hyperorality and dietary changes
- perseverative and stereotyped behaviour
- utilization behaviour

READINGS AND REFERENCES
Neary D, Snowden JS, Gustafson L, et al. Frontotemporal lobar degeneration: a consensus on clinical diagnostic criteria. *Neurology*. 1998;51(6):1546–1554. Medline:9855500

11. **Which of the following findings is true about dementia with Lewy bodies (DLB)?**
   a. It is more prevalent in females.
   b. Lewy bodies are eosinophilic extra cytoplasmic inclusion bodies.
   c. Early loss of language is common.
   d. Extrapyramidal symptoms (EPS) are reported in 25% to 50% of DLB cases.
   e. Patients with DLB generally perform poorly on tests of verbal memory.

Answer: d

DLB is a common form of senile dementia, and shares clinical and pathological features with both Alzheimer disease and Parkinson disease. However, its neuropsychological impairments are different, indicating a combined involvement of cortical and subcortical pathways. It is more common in males than females, and it is an underdiagnosed condition. Language is preserved until late disease stages. Lewy bodies are eosinophilic intracytoplasmic neuronal inclusions of abnormally phosphorylated neurofilament proteins.

Compared with Alzheimer patients, DLB patients generally perform better on tests of verbal memory, but worse on visuospatial performance tasks. Extrapyramidal symptoms are commonly reported (25% to 50% of cases) and almost 80% of patients develop some EPS during the course of the illness.

READINGS AND REFERENCES
McKeith IG. Dementia with Lewy bodies. In: Agronin ME, Maletta GJ. *Principles and Practice of Geriatric Psychiatry.* 2nd ed. Philadelphia: Wolters Kluwer/Lippincott Williams & Wilkins; 2011:334–335.

Weiner MF. Dementia associated with Lewy bodies: dilemmas and directions *Arch Neurol*. 1999;56(12):1441–1442. Medline:10593296

12. Which of the following findings is not seen in normal pressure hydrocephalus (NPH)?

a. ataxia
b. urinary incontinence
c. irreversible dementia
d. normal cerebrospinal fluid pressure
e. progressive slowing of cognitive function

Answer: c

NPH patients have dilated cerebral ventricles (third ventricle) and normal cerebrospinal fluid (CSF) pressure. The classic triad of symptoms is gait ataxia, dementia, and urinary incontinence (late symptom). NPH is potentially reversible if treated promptly.

READINGS AND REFERENCES
Shprecher D, Schwalb J, Kurlan R. Normal pressure hydrocephalus: diagnosis and treatment. *Curr Neurol Neurosci Rep.* 2008;8(5):371–376. Medline:18713572

13. Which of the following statements is true about cortical dementia compared to subcortical dementia?

a. slowed cognitive processing
b. prominent psychomotor retardation
c. gait disturbance
d. severe depression
e. significant memory impairment

Answer: e

The following features favour cortical dementia over subcortical dementia:
- significant memory impairment
- aphasia, apraxia, and agnosia
- executive dysfunction
- late onset and less prominent motor disturbances

In addition:
- Apathy is less common in cortical dementia than in subcortical dementia.
- Depression is less prominent in cortical dementia than in subcortical dementia.

READINGS AND REFERENCES
Lavretsky H, Chui H. Vascular dementia. In: Agronin ME, Maletta GJ, eds. *Principles and Practice of Geriatric Psychiatry*. 2nd edition. Philadelphia: Wolters Kluwer/Lippincott Williams & Wilkins; 2011:321.

14. **Which of the following rating scales is used in assessing externalizing behaviours?**
    a. Child Behavior Checklist (CBCL)
    b. Conners Rating Scale
    c. Mania Rating Scale
    d. Beck Depression Inventory
    e. Children's Depression Rating Scale

Answer: b

Broad-band rating scales are not specific to particular diagnoses or constructs, but can assess multiple dimensions of problematic and adaptive behaviour. Some commonly used broad-band scales are the Child Behaviour Checklist (CBCL) and Youth Self-Report (YSR).

Symptoms of attention-deficit/hyperactivity disorder, oppositional defiant disorder, and conduct disorders are assessed with rating scales that evaluate externalizing behaviours—i.e., ADHD-IV scale, Conners rating scale, Home Situations Questionnaires (HSQ). Rating scales such as the Beck Depression Inventory (BDI) and Hamilton Depression Rating Scale (HAM-D) are used in assessing depression and anxiety.

READINGS AND REFERENCES
Myers K, Collett B. Rating scales. In: Dulcan M, Wiener J, eds. *Essentials of Child and Adolescent Psychiatry*. Arlington, VA: American Psychiatric Publishing; 2006:83–86.

15. **Which of the following syndromes is not correctly paired with its chromosomal abnormality?**
    a. Prader-Willi syndrome: deletion of chromosome 15 of paternal origin
    b. fragile X syndrome: fragile site on the long (q) arm of the X chromosome at Xq27.3
    c. cri du chat syndrome: deletion of chromosome at 5p15.2 of paternal origin
    d. Down syndrome: trisomy 18
    e. Angelman syndrome: deletion within 15q11q13 of maternal origin

Answer: d

Down syndrome is caused by primary nondisjunction leading to trisomy 21.

In Prader-Willi syndrome, about 70% of those affected have a deletion on the long arm of chromosome 15 (del 15q11q13). The deleted chromosome is always of paternal origin.

Fragile X syndrome is an X-linked disorder. A fragile site on the long (q) arm of the X chromosome at Xq27.3, and the "fragility" of the X chromosome, is now known to be associated with an unstable region of DNA within the fragile X mental retardation 1 (FMR1) gene.

Cri du chat syndrome is thought to be associated with deletions in 5p15.2 of paternal origin. Most of the deletions are spontaneous. About 15% of affected people have an unbalanced translocation and a small number of cases (1%) are due to inherited deletions.

Angelman syndrome is caused by a deletion within 15q11q13 of maternal origin. It is also occasionally associated with paternal uniparental disomy, but this is less common than in Prader-Willi syndrome.

READINGS AND REFERENCES
Clarke DM, Deb S. Syndromes causing intellectual disability. In: Gelder MG, Andreasen MD, López-Ibor JJ Jr, Geddes R, eds. *New Oxford Textbook of Psychiatry*. Vol 2. 2nd ed. Oxford: Oxford University Press; 2012:1839–1844.

16. Which of the following is true of patients who have early onset bipolar disorder?

a. They have higher rates of psychotic features than those with onset at an older age.
b. Early onset of symptoms indicates a shorter course of illness.
c. Children with bipolar disorder are more responsive to treatment than adults.
d. Grandiose delusions are more common than paranoid delusions.
e. Euphoria is more common than irritability and unpredictable mood.

Answer: a

Patients who have early onset bipolar disorder have: higher rates of psychotic features; a more severe course of illness; significant behaviour disorder in childhood; poor school performance; more frequent substance-use disorder at the onset of their mood disorder; more paranoid features to their presentation; and excessive grandiosity. In early onset bipolar disorder, irritability and an unpredictable and labile mood are more common than euphoria.

READINGS AND REFERENCES
Ballenger JC, Reus VI, Post RM. The "atypical" clinical picture of adolescent mania. *Am J Psychiatry*. 1982;139(5):602–606. Medline:7072845
Joyce PR. Age of onset in bipolar affective disorder and misdiagnosis as schizophrenia. *Psychol Med*. 1984;14(1):145–149. Medline:6709780
McElroy SL, Strakowski SM, West SA, et al. Phenomenology of adolescent and adult mania in hospitalized patients with bipolar disorder. *Am J Psychiatry*. 1997;154(1):44–49. Medline:8988957
McGlashan TH. Adolescent versus adult onset of mania. *Am J Psychiatry*. 1988;145(2):221–223. Medline:3124634
Weller EB, Kloos AL, Weller RA. Mood disorders. In: Dulcan M, Wiener J, eds. *Essentials of Child and Adolescent Psychiatry*. Arlington, VA: American Psychiatric Publishing; 2006:273–274.

17. Mothers of children diagnosed with conduct disorder are more likely to have which of the following conditions?
 a. somatization
 b. criminal behaviour
 c. anxiety disorders
 d. depression
 e. bipolar disorder

Answer: a

Parental psychopathology has a strong association with conduct disorder in children. Mothers of children diagnosed with conduct disorder often have antisocial personality, somatization, or problems with alcohol abuse. Antisocial personality disorder, criminal behaviour, and alcoholism—particularly in the father—are stronger and more consistently reported familial factors that increase children's risk for conduct disorder.

READINGS AND REFERENCES

Hendren RL, Mullen DJ. Conduct disorder and oppositional defiant disorder. In: Dulcan M, Wiener J. *Essentials of Child and Adolescent Psychiatry*. Arlington, VA: American Psychiatric Publishing; 2006:357–385.

Lahey BB, Piacentini JC, McBurnett K, Stone P, Hartdagen S, Hynd G. Psychopathology in the parents of children with conduct disorder and hyperactivity. *J Am Acad Child Adolesc Psychiatry*. 1988;27(2):163-70. Medline:3360717

Robins, LN. *Deviant Children Grown Up*. Baltimore, MD: Williams and Wilkins; 1966.

Rutter M, Giller H. *Juvenile Delinquency: Trends and Perspectives*. Harmondsworth, UK: Penguin; 1983.

18. Which of the following is true about Tourette syndrome?
 a. Both multiple and 1 or more vocal tics should be present.
 b. Coprolalia is a common early symptom.
 c. It is more common in girls.
 d. It is usually associated with psychotic symptoms.
 e. Treatment with D_2 receptor antagonists usually completely suppresses the tics.

Answer: a

DSM-5 specifies that in Tourette syndrome "both multiple and 1 or more vocal tics should be present at some time during the illness, although not necessarily concurrently."

Tourette syndrome is 4 times more common in boys and the onset is before age 18. Young age of onset is associated with more severe tics. Prevalence is 5 to 30 in 10 000. Treatment is usually with D_2 receptor antagonists such as haloperidol, or with atypical antipsychotics including risperidone, aripiprazole, and quetiapine.

READINGS AND REFERENCES

American Psychiatric Association. *Diagnostic and Statistical Manual of Mental Disorders.* 5th ed. Washington, DC: American Psychiatric Publishing; 2013:81.

Schlesinger AB, Horner MS, Malley E, et al. Child and adolescent psychiatry. In: Kupfer DJ, Horner MS, Brent DA, et al, eds. *Oxford American Handbook of Psychiatry.* Oxford: Oxford University Press; 2008:748–749.

19. Which of the following author-theory pairings is correct?

a. Rogers: object relations theory
b. Klein: transactional analysis
c. Berne: client centred therapy
d. Erikson: alternative model of psychosocial development
e. Winnicot: theories of childhood development, including primitive defence mechanisms such as splitting

Answer: d

The following authors and theories are correctly paired:

- Carl Rogers: client centred therapy
- Melanie Klein: theories of childhood development, including primitive defence mechanism
- Eric Berne: transactional analysis
- Erik Erikson: alternative model of psychosocial development
- Donald Winnicot: object relation theory

READINGS AND REFERENCES

Sadock BJ, Sadock VA. *Kaplan and Sadock's Synopsis of Psychiatry: Behavioral Sciences/Clinical Psychiatry.* 10th ed. Philadelphia: Wolters Kluwer/Lippincott Williams & Wilkins; 2007:214–226.

20. Which of the following is not a characteristic test for frontal lobe function?

a. Category Fluency Test
b. Go-No-Go task
c. Cognitive Estimate Test
d. reproducing interlocking pentagons
e. Luria test

Answer: d

Reproducing interlocking pentagons assesses visuospatial skills. Other tasks (during a mini–mental state examination) that assess visuospatial skills include drawing a clock face with numbers, and drawing 3-dimensional objects, such as a wire cube. Deficits in visuospatial skills are seen in neurodegenerative diseases, particularly Alzheimer disease.

The other tests listed in this question assess frontal lobe function. Patients with frontal lobe pathology respond to these tests as follows:
- Go-No-Go tasks: impulsive decisions (which are thought to show failure of response inhibition and frontal lobe pathology)
- Cognitive Estimate Test: bizarre or improbable answers (e.g., patients may drastically over- or underestimate the population of their town or city)
- Category Fluency Test: impaired response (e.g., a normal response to "name as many animals as possible in 1 minute" is 20 animals; 15 is low average; fewer than 10 is impaired)
- Luria test: impaired response (e.g., patients are unable to perform an assigned sequence of motor activities, which is thought to be a frontal lobe task)

READINGS AND REFERENCES
Kipps CM, Hodges JR. Clinical cognitive assessment. In: Jacoby R, Oppenheimer C, Dening T, Thomas A, eds. *Oxford Textbook of Old Age Psychiatry*. Oxford: Oxford University Press; 2008:159–160, 161.

21. Which of the following neuroimaging findings does not indicate vascular dementia?
a. ischemic infarction
b. subcortical vascular encephalopathy
c. fornix infarcts
d. amyloid angiopathy
e. bilateral thalamic hyperintensity

Answer: e

Bilateral thalamic hyperintensity in T_2 proton-weighted images due to a thalamic gliosis—the "pulvinar sign"—is associated with Creutzfeldt-Jacob disease.

All the other findings listed in this question are seen in vascular dementia.

READINGS AND REFERENCES
Hentschel F, Förstl H. Neuroimaging and neurophysiology in the elderly. In: Jacoby R, Oppenheimer C, Dening T, Thomas A, eds. *Oxford Textbook of Old Age Psychiatry*. Oxford: Oxford University Press; 2008:181–187.

22. Which of the following statements is true about cholinesterase inhibitors?
a. Galantamine is an irreversible competitive inhibitor of acetylcholinesterase.
b. Memantine is effective in mild Alzheimer disease.
c. The effects of cholinesterase inhibitors on behavioural disturbances are dose dependent.

d. Donepezil is an irreversible inhibitor of acetylcholinesterase.

   e. Rivastigmine is a pseudo-irreversible inhibitor of acetylcholinesterase.

Answer: e

Rivastigmine increases the concentration of acetylcholine through reversible inhibition of its hydrolysis by cholinesterase. It can be categorized as a noncompetitive, pseudo-irreversible cholinesterase inhibitor due to its prolonged enzyme inhibition activity.

Galantamine, a tertiary alkaloid, is a competitive and reversible inhibitor of acetylcholinesterase.

Memantine is indicated for severe Alzheimer-type dementia, but not for mild cases.

The effects of cholinesterase inhibitors on cognition and functional activities are dose dependent, but effects on behavioural disturbances are not.

Donepezil is a reversible inhibitor of acetylcholinesterase.

READINGS AND REFERENCES

Virani AS, Bezchlibnyk-Butler KZ, Jeffries JJ, Procyshyn RM, eds. *Clinical Handbook of Psychotropic Drugs*. 19th ed. Cambridge, MA: Hogrefe Publishing; 2012:236–243.

Wilcock G. Clinical aspects of dementia: specific pharmacological treatments for Alzheimer's disease. In: Jacoby R, Oppenheimer C, Dening T, Thomas A, eds. *Oxford Textbook of Old Age Psychiatry*. Oxford: Oxford University Press; 2008:483–487.

23. Which of the following is true about sleep changes in elderly patients (older than 65)?

   a. shorter sleep latency

   b. shorter rapid eye movement (REM) latency

   c. increased total sleep time

   d. less stage 1 and 2 sleep

   e. more slow-wave sleep

Answer: b

The following sleep changes are seen in elderly patients:
- reduced total sleep time
- more daytime napping
- reduced percentage of REM sleep
- longer arousal periods
- more frequent arousal periods
- transitory and perceptual phenomena in the borders of sleep (common)

READINGS AND REFERENCES

Morsimann UP, Boeve BF. Sleep disorders in older people. In: Jacoby R, Oppenheimer C, Dening T, Thomas A, eds. *Oxford Textbook of Old Age Psychiatry*. Oxford: Oxford University Press; 2008:673–675.

24. Which of the following is not a characteristic of a positive family history for alcoholism?
a. family history of depression
b. conduct disorder during childhood
c. deficit in executive cognitive functioning
d. attention-deficit/hyperactivity disorder (ADHD) as a child
e. low educational achievement

Answer: a

Except for family history of depression, all the other answers in this question are characteristics of familial alcoholism.

READINGS AND REFERENCES
Negrete JC, Gill K. Aetiology of alcohol problems. In: Gelder MG, Andreasen MD, López-Ibor JJ Jr, Geddes R, eds. *New Oxford Textbook of Psychiatry*. Vol 1. 2nd ed. Oxford, UK: Oxford University Press; 2012:432–437.

25. A meta-analysis of published and unpublished randomized control trials of antidepressants assessed the number needed to treat (NNT) to achieve benefits from antidepressants. The antidepressants studied were selective serotonin reuptake inhibitors (SSRIs) and serotonin-norepinephrine reuptake inhibitors (SNRIs). What value did the study find for the NNT?
a. 5%
b. 10%
c. 15%
d. 20%
e. 25%

Answer: b

NNT is defined as the number of patients who must receive treatment to get one response that is attributable to the active treatment.

READINGS AND REFERENCES
Bridge JA, Iyengar S, Salary CB, et al. Clinical response and risk for reported suicidal ideation and suicide attempts in pediatric antidepressant treatment: a meta-analysis of randomized controlled trials. *JAMA*. 2007;297(15);1683–1696. Medline:17440145

26. The US National Institute of Mental Health (NIMH) conducted a study of methylphenidate among 3- to 5-year-olds: the Preschool ADHD Treatment Study (PATS). Which of the following is not a finding of the study?
a. Methylphenidate is effective in preschoolers with ADHD.
b. Eleven percent of subjects withdrew from the study because of adverse events.

c. Methylphenidate resulted in lower rates of emotional adverse events (e.g., irritability and crying episodes) in the study group compared to older children.
d. The mean optimal dose of methylphenidate was lower than the mean optimal dose for school-age children.
e. Preschoolers metabolized methylphenidate slower than school-age children.

Answer: c

The NIMH-sponsored PATS is a major study of preschoolers with ADHD. It involved 183 children who underwent an open-label trial of methylphenidate. Of these children, 165 were randomized into a 6-week double-blinded, placebo-controlled crossover trial of methylphenidate. This study showed that these children were more irritable and more prone to crying episodes compared to older children.

READINGS AND REFERENCES
Greenhill LL, Kollins S, Abikoff H, et al. Efficacy and safety of immediate-release methylphenidate treatment for preschoolers with ADHD. *J Am Acad Child Adolesc Psychiatry*. 2006;45(11):1284–1293. Medline:17023867

McGough J, McCracken J, Swanson J, et al. Pharmacogenetics of methylphenidate response in preschoolers with ADHD. *J Am Acad Child Adolesc Psychiatry*. 2006;45(11):1314–1322. Medline:17023870

27. A major US study of therapies for pediatric obsessive-compulsive disorder—the Pediatric OCD Treatment Study (POTS)—evaluated the acute efficacy of sertraline, cognitive behavioural therapy (CBT), combination treatment (CBT and sertraline), and placebo. Which of the following statements is not a conclusion of the study?
    a. Response to CBT, sertraline, and combination treatment was significantly greater than placebo.
    b. Response to combination treatment was superior to CBT or sertraline alone.
    c. The remission rate for combination treatment was lower compared to sertraline, CBT, or placebo.
    d. The remission rate for sertraline was not different from placebo.
    e. The remission rate for CBT was not different from sertraline, but was greater than placebo.

Answer: c

The POTS showed remission rates were:
- 53.6% (95% CI*: 36%–70%) for combination treatment
- 39.3% (95% CI: 24%–58%) for CBT

- 21.4% (95% CI: 10%–40%) for sertraline
- 3.6% (95% CI: 0%–19%) for placebo

The study recommends that adolescents with OCD start treatment with combination treatment or CBT alone.

READINGS AND REFERENCES
Pediatric OCD Treatment Study Team. Cognitive behavior therapy, sertraline and their combination for children and adolescents with obsessive-compulsive disorder: the Pediatric OCD Treatment Study (POTS) randomized controlled trial. *JAMA.* 2004;292(16):1969–1976. Medline:15507582

28. Benzodiazepines are used for anxiety disorders. Which of the following statements is not true regarding the mechanism of action of benzodiazepines?
    a. Benzodiazepine receptors appear to be part of the membrane complexes involving chloride channels and GABA receptors.
    b. At these sites, benzodiazepines bind to larger protein complexes found on the receptors and facilitate $GABA_B$ transmission, which leads to increased chloride conductance and increased inhibition of the central nervous system (CNS).
    c. Benzodiazepines lower serotonin turnover and activity.
    d. Benzodiazepines lower the spontaneous firing of noradrenergic neurons in the locus coeruleus.
    e. Benzodiazepines decrease dopaminergic function.

Answer: b

Benzodiazepines facilitate $GABA_A$ transmission. They also exhibit diffuse inhibitory effects on the CNS. The facilitation of GABAergic transmission and CNS-function inhibition are believed to directly produce the anxiolytic, sedative, hypnotic, and anticonvulsant and muscle-relaxant properties of this group of medications.

READINGS AND REFERENCES
Coffey BJ, Zwilling AL. Anxiolytics. In: Rosenberg DR, Gershon S, eds. *Pharmacotherapy of Child and Adolescent Psychiatric Disorders.* 3rd ed. Chichester, UK: Wiley-Blackwell; 2012:301–340.

29. Because of the possible cardiac effects of stimulants, physicians need to check the personal and family history of children and adolescents before treating them with stimulants. Which of the following is not relevant in this context?
    a. tetralogy of Fallot
    b. cardiac artery abnormalities
    c. obstructive subaortic stenosis

d. edema of the lower extremities
e. previous consultation with a cardiologist

Answer: d

Physicians should have a thorough discussion with patients and their families about the cardiac-related risks of stimulants. Physicians should ask about personal or family history of structural cardiac disorders. They should also determine if patients have hypertension, arrhythmias, chest pain, or symptoms of syncope; these may indicate hypertrophic cardiomyopathy, a condition associated with sudden death in patients taking stimulants.

READINGS AND REFERENCES
Pliszka SR. Psychostimulants. In: Rosenberg DR, Gershon S, eds. *Pharmacotherapy of Child and Adolescent Psychiatric Disorders*. 3rd ed. Chichester, UK: Wiley-Blackwell; 2012:65–104.

30. Which of the following statements about mood stabilizers is true?
    a. Carbamazepine doses need to be increased when used in combination with valproate.
    b. Valproate doubles lamotrigine levels when used in combination, so dosing should be one-half that of normal.
    c. Carbamazepine is a weak 3A4 inducer.
    d. Inhibition of 3A4 will notably decrease carbamazepine levels.
    e. Carbamazepine increases levels of haloperidol when used in combination.

Answer: b

Carbamazepine doses need to be decreased when used in combination with valproate. Carbamazepine is a potent 3A4 inducer. The inhibition of 3A4 notably increases carbamazepine levels. Carbamazepine decreases the levels of haloperidol when used in combination.

READINGS AND REFERENCES
Post R. Lithium and related mood stabilizers. In: Gelder MG, Andreasen MD, López-Ibor JJ Jr, Geddes R, eds. *New Oxford Textbook of Psychiatry*. Vol 2. 2nd ed. Oxford, UK: Oxford University Press; 2012:1199–1207.

31. Which of the following statements is true about brief psychotic disorder?
    a. The average age of onset is mid-20s.
    b. Symptoms last at least 1 day but not longer than 1 week.
    c. It is twice as common in females.
    d. Paranoid personality disorder is a risk factor for developing brief psychotic disorder.
    e. The outcome is usually poor due to difficulties in social functioning.

Answer: c

According to *DSM-5*, brief psychotic disorder has the following characteristics:
- onset: it can occur across the life span; average age of onset is mid-30s
- duration: episodes last at least 1 day, but less than 1 month
- outcome: individuals have full return to premorbid level of functioning within 1 month of onset
- risk factors: preexisting personality disorders and traits may predispose individuals to brief psychotic disorder—e.g., schizotypal personality disorder; borderline personality disorder; traits in the psychoticism domain (e.g., perceptual dysregulations); traits in the negative affectivity domain (e.g., suspiciousness)

READINGS AND REFERENCES
American Psychiatric Association. *Diagnostic and Statistical Manual of Mental Disorders.* 5th ed. Washington, DC: American Psychiatric Publishing; 2013:94–96.

32. Which of the following brain regions is involved in OCD?
a. amygdala
b. cerebellum
c. basal ganglia
d. hypothalamus
e. locus coeruleus

Answer: c

Positron emission tomography has shown that patients with OCD have increased metabolism and blood flow in the:
- frontal lobes
- basal ganglia (especially the caudate nucleus)
- cingulum

Pharmacological and behavioural treatments reportedly reverse these abnormalities.

READINGS AND REFERENCES
Baxter LR, Schwartz JM, Bergman KS, et al. Caudate glucose metabolic rate changes with both drug and behavior therapy for obsessive-compulsive disorder. *Arch Gen Psychiatry.* 1992;49(9):681–689. Medline:1514872.

Gilbert AR, MacPhee ER, Gilbert AM. Anxiety and stress-related disorders. In: Kupfer DJ, Horner MS, Brent DA, et al, eds. *Oxford American Handbook of Psychiatry.* Oxford: Oxford University Press; 2008:422.

Rauch, S.L. Neuroimaging in OCD: clinical implications. *CNS Spectrums.* 1998;3(suppl 1):26–29.

Sadock BJ, Sadock VA. *Kaplan and Sadock's Comprehensive Textbook of Psychiatry: Behavioral Sciences/Clinical Psychiatry*. 9th ed. Philadelphia: Wolters Kluwer/Lippincott Williams & Wilkins; 2009:3671–3678.

33. Which of the following statements about gabapentin is true?
a. It exerts its effects through direct regulation of benzodiazepine receptors.
b. It has a benign drug-interaction profile with no active metabolites.
c. It has significant cytochrome P450 interactions.
d. It acts as a GABA precursor.
e. It has excellent protein-binding capacity.

Answer: b

The mechanism of gabapentin is not fully understood, but it is thought to block voltage-dependent sodium channels and calcium channels. It was originally developed as an analogue of GABA, the major inhibitory neurotransmitter in the cerebral cortex. It has a benign drug-interaction profile with no active metabolites and is eliminated by renal excretion. It has no plasma protein-binding or cytochrome P450 interactions. It does not act as a GABA precursor.

READINGS AND REFERENCES
Virani AS, Bezchlibnyk-Butler KZ, Jeffries JJ, Procyshyn RM, eds. *Clinical Handbook of Psychotropic Drugs*. 18th ed. Cambridge, MA: Hogrefe Publishing; 2009:197–199.

34. Which of the following is true about culture-bound disorders?
a. Koro is mostly associated with Mexico.
b. Windigo involves fear of engaging in cannibalism.
c. Latah is the belief that the penis will retract into the abdomen and cause death.
d. Amok has a history in Malaysia and is an anxiety-associated condition.
e. Automatic obedience hypersuggestibility is seen in frigophobia.

Answer: b

Windigo has a history with Canadian First Nations peoples, and is fear of engaging in cannibalism and of becoming a sorcerer.

Koro is known worldwide by various names. It is most commonly seen in Malaysia and South Asia. It involves fear that the genitals are retracting into the abdomen and will result in death.

Latah has a history in Southeast Asia and involves hypersensitivity to startle, often in association with echopraxia, echolalia, command obedience, and trancelike behaviour.

Amok is a dissociative state with a history in Malaysia, Laos, Philippines, and South Asia. The condition involves automatism, amnesia, and exhaustion. Individuals—who are usually younger, male, and living away from home—recover to a premorbid state.

Frigophobia has a history in East Asia. It involves morbid fear of the cold, preoccupation with loss of vitality, and compulsive wearing of multiple layers of clothing.

READINGS AND REFERENCES

Sadock BJ, Sadock VA. *Kaplan and Sadock's Synopsis of Psychiatry: Behavioral Sciences/ Clinical Psychiatry*. 9th ed. Philadelphia: Wolters Kluwer/Lippincott Williams & Wilkins; 2003:2523–2524.

Sims, A. *Symptoms in the Mind: An Introduction to Descriptive Psychopathology*. 2nd ed. Edinburgh: Saunders; 1995:238.

35. **Which of the following statements is true about speech disturbances associated with schizophrenia?**

   a. logoclonia

   b. stuttering

   c. dysarthria

   d. cryptolalia

   e. aphonia

Answer: d

Unintelligible speech (e.g., neologisms, stock words and phrases), cryptographia, and cryptolalia may occur in schizophrenia.

Logoclonia is the spastic repetition of syllables that occurs in parkinsonism: the patient may get stuck using a particular word.

Stuttering is not seen in schizophrenia.

Dysarthria is disorder of articulation that impairs the mechanism of phonation. It is seen in lesions of the brain stem (stroke) and schizophrenia.

Aphonia is a loss of the ability to vocalize; patients talk by whispering.

READINGS AND REFERENCES

Sims, A. *Symptoms in the Mind: An Introduction to Descriptive Psychopathology*. 2nd ed. Edinburgh: Saunders; 1995:158–159.

36. **Which of the following is true of depressive disorder with melancholic features?**

   a. hypersomnia

   b. significant anorexia

   c. leaden paralysis

   d. mood reactivity

   e. affective flattening

Answer: b

According to *DSM-5*, depressive disorder with melancholic features has 1 of the following symptoms during the most severe period of the current episode:
- loss of pleasure in all or almost all activities
- lack of reactivity to usually pleasurable stimuli

Three or more of the following are also present:
- excessive or inappropriate guilt
- significant anorexia or weight loss
- marked psychomotor retardation or agitation
- early morning awakening
- depression that is regularly worse in the morning
- empty mood

This is different from depressive disorder with atypical features, which is distinguished by:
- mood reactivity
- 2 or more of the following: weight gain, hypersomnia, leaden paralysis, long-standing interpersonal rejection sensitivity

READINGS AND REFERENCES
American Psychiatric Association. *Diagnostic and Statistical Manual of Mental Disorders.* 5th ed. Washington, DC: American Psychiatric Publishing; 2013:185–186.

37. Which of the following symptoms is suggestive of delirium rather than dementia?
    a. insidious onset
    b. progressive course
    c. fixed delusions
    d. incongruity of mood
    e. labile affect

Answer: e

Delirium is typically characterized by:
- acute onset
- fluctuating course
- reversibility (frequently)
- impaired level of consciousness
- inattention and labile affect (common)

Delusions are fleeting, fragmented, and usually persecutory. They often relate to the immediate environment or impending danger.

READINGS AND REFERENCES
Trzepacz P, Meagher D. Delirium. In: Gelder MG, Andreasen MD, López-Ibor JJ Jr, Geddes R, eds. *New Oxford Textbook of Psychiatry*. Vol 1. 2nd ed. Oxford, UK: Oxford University Press; 2012:328.

38. Which of the following is a sign of acute phencyclidine intoxication?

a. hypotension
b. bradycardia
c. pinpoint pupils
d. nystagmus
e. respiratory arrest with a pulse

Answer: d

DSM-5 lists the following as criteria for phencyclidine intoxication: agitation; belligerence; impaired judgment; vertical or horizontal nystagmus; hyperacusis; hypertension or tachycardia; numbness; ataxia; dysarthria; rigidity; and seizure or coma.

Opioid overdose is associated with hypotension, bradycardia, pinpoint pupils, and respiratory arrest with a pulse.

READINGS AND REFERENCES
American Psychiatric Association. *Diagnostic and Statistical Manual of Mental Disorders*. 5th ed. Washington, DC: American Psychiatric Publishing; 2013:528–529.

39. Which of the following antidepressants is associated with fewer sexual side effects?

a. bupropion
b. paroxetine
c. venlafaxine
d. fluoxetine
e. fluvoxamine

Answer: a

All SSRIs and SNRIs are associated with significant sexual side effects. The common side effects are decreased libido, impotence, ejaculatory disturbances, anorgasmia, and delayed orgasm. Bupropion rarely impairs sexual functioning and in some cases improvement is noted.

READINGS AND REFERENCES
Taylor M, Rudkin L, Hawton K. Strategies for managing antidepressant-induced sexual dysfunction: systematic review of randomised controlled trials. *Journal of Affective Disorders*. 2005;88(3):241–254. Medline:16162361
Virani AS, Bezchlibnyk-Butler KZ, Jeffries JJ, Procyshyn RM, eds. *Clinical Handbook of Psychotropic Drugs*. 18th ed. Cambridge, MA: Hogrefe Publishing; 2009:2–16.

40. A 70-year old man presents with worsening forgetfulness and is unable to keep his appointments. Which of the following would suggest a mild cognitive impairment in this patient?
   a. evidence of significant cortical dysfunction
   b. changes in his activities of daily living
   c. objective memory impairment for his age
   d. evidence suggestive of dementia
   e. changes in mood

Answer: c

The following would suggest mild cognitive impairment:
- memory complaint, preferably confirmed by an informant
- no impairment in activities of daily living
- objective memory impairment for age
- no evidence of dementia
- normal general cognition

READINGS AND REFERENCES
American Psychiatric Association. *Diagnostic and Statistical Manual of Mental Disorders.* 5th ed. Washington, DC: American Psychiatric Publishing; 2013:605–611.

41. Which of the following is a protective factor against persistence of violence?
   a. being last-born
   b. coming from a large family
   c. being an active and affective infant
   d. low intelligence quotient (IQ)
   e. exposure to parental conflict

Answer: c

The following are protective factors against persistence of violence:
- being first-born
- coming from a small family
- resilient temperament
- high IQ
- receiving a large amount of attention from caregivers
- prosocial relationships with peers, family, and teachers

READINGS AND REFERENCES
Eastman N, Adshead G, Fox S, et al. *Forensic Psychiatry.* Oxford Specialist Handbooks in Psychiatry. Oxford: Oxford University Press; 2012:53–88.

42. Which of the following factors is not associated with poor prognosis in anorexia nervosa?
    a. older age of onset
    b. longer duration of illness
    c. personality problems
    d. good family support
    e. bulimic features

Answer: d

Death from anorexia nervosa is more likely in women, and suicide rates are high. Good family support is associated with good prognosis.

READINGS AND REFERENCES
Marcus MD, Wilson DV. Eating and impulse control disorders. In: Kupfer DJ, Horner MS, Brent DA, et al, eds. *Oxford American Handbook of Psychiatry*. Oxford: Oxford University Press; 2008:457.

43. Which of the following conditions should not be considered in the differential diagnosis of a patient with body dysmorphic disorder?
    a. major depressive disorder
    b. obsessive-compulsive personality disorder (OCPD)
    c. schizophrenia
    d. social phobia
    e. trichotillomania

Answer: b

Body dysmorphic disorder is closely related to obsessive-compulsive and related disorders. No evidence suggests, however, that it is connected with OCPD.

All the other answers listed for this question should be considered in the differential diagnosis for body dysmorphic disorder.

READINGS AND REFERENCES
American Psychiatric Association. *Diagnostic and Statistical Manual of Mental Disorders*. 5th ed. Washington, DC; 2013:242–247,678–682.

44. According to the Social Readjustment Rating Scale, which of the following life changes is considered highly stressful?
    a. death of a spouse
    b. divorce
    c. retirement from work
    d. death of a close family member
    e. detention in jail

Answer: a

Life events are associated with psychiatric disorders. Thomas Holmes and Richard Rahe constructed the Social Readjustment Rating Scale to measure the impact of life events. According to their study, death of a spouse is most stressful, followed by divorce, detention in jail, and death of a close family member.

READINGS AND REFERENCES

Holmes TH. Life situations, emotions, and disease. *Psychosomatics*. 1978; 19(12): 747–754. Medline:734029

Sadock BJ, Sadock VA. *Kaplan and Sadock's Synopsis of Psychiatry: Behavioral Sciences/Clinical Psychiatry*. 10th ed. Philadelphia: Wolters Kluwer/Lippincott Williams & Wilkins; 2007:815.

45. Which of the following statements about brief focal psychotherapy is true?
    a. Resolution of the Oedipus complex is part of the therapy.
    b. Duration is 12 treatment hours.
    c. Challenging defenses is the primary focus of therapy.
    d. Catharsis is promoted.
    e. Linking the past, the present, and the transference is important.

Answer: e

In brief focal psychotherapy, the goal is to clarify the nature of the defence, the anxiety, and the impulse. It usually lasts up to 1 year and focuses on internal conflicts present since childhood.

Resolution of the Oedipus conflict is part of short-term anxiety-provoking therapy.

READINGS AND REFERENCES

Sadock BJ, Sadock VA. *Kaplan and Sadock's Synopsis of Psychiatry: Behavioral Sciences/Clinical Psychiatry*. 10th ed. Philadelphia: Wolters Kluwer/Lippincott Williams & Wilkins; 2007:932–933.

46. Which of the following statements about neuroleptic malignant syndrome (NMS) is true?
    a. The onset of NMS is rapid.
    b. Hyperkinesia is seen.
    c. NMS progresses rapidly.
    d. Muscle rigidity is commonly seen.
    e. NMS is more common in women.

Answer: d

NMS is slow in onset; symptoms progress slowly over 24 to 72 hours. Men are affected more than women, and younger individuals more than older individuals. The mortality rate is high: 10% to 20%. The symptoms include: muscle rigidity; dystonia; akinesia or bradykinesia; mutism; obtundation; and agitation. Autonomic symptoms are also common (e.g., high fever, sweating, increased pulse, increased blood pressure).

READINGS AND REFERENCES
Sadock BJ, Sadock VA. *Kaplan and Sadock's Synopsis of Psychiatry: Behavioral Sciences/ Clinical Psychiatry*. 10th ed. Philadelphia: Wolters Kluwer/Lippincott Williams & Wilkins; 2007:995.

47. Which of the following symptoms is most commonly seen in patients with PTSD?
    a. anxiety at reminders of the trauma
    b. recurrent nightmares
    c. insomnia
    d. restricted affect
    e. increased use of alcohol

Answer: c

According to a study by Green, insomnia is the most common symptom of patients with PTSD, followed by anxiety at reminders of the trauma, intrusive thoughts, poor concentration, and irritability.

READINGS AND REFERENCES
Green B. Post-traumatic stress disorder: symptom profiles in men and women. *Curr Med Res Opin*. 2003;19(3):200–204. Medline:12803734

48. Which of the following is true about cardiovascular changes associated with aging?
    a. increase in heart size
    b. increase in flexibility of the collagen matrix
    c. fat destruction in the myocardium
    d. increased left ventricular diastolic filling
    e. reduced peak exercise index and ejection fraction

Answer: e

Several physiologic changes occur in the process of aging including: changes in the heart and blood vessels; decrease in cardiac output and cardiac reserve; thickening of blood vessels; increase in systolic blood pressure; left ventricular enlargement; decrease in cardiac output; and decrease in maximum oxygen consumption.

READINGS AND REFERENCES
Blazer DG, Steffens DC. *Essentials of Geriatric Psychiatry*. 2nd ed. Arlington, VA: American Psychiatric Publishing; 2012:31.

49. Which of the following statements is true about the use of neuroleptics for OCD?

a. First-generation neuroleptics are usually helpful.

b. Second-generation agents such as risperidone can be used as monotherapy.

c. Neuroleptics may worsen OCD symptoms if used without an SSRI.

d. Neuroleptics are the primary choice of treatment for OCD.

e. For ODC patients, neuroleptics act more quickly than SSRIs.

Answer: c

First-generation neuroleptics are rarely helpful in OCD. They are helpful as augmenting agents in OCD patients who also have tics.

Second-generation antipsychotics can be combined with SSRIs; they are generally not used as first-line agents.

SSRIs are the treatment of choice for OCD.

READINGS AND REFERENCES

DeVeaugh-Geiss J, Landeau P, Katz R. Preliminary results from a multicenter trial of clomipramine in obsessive-compulsive disorder. *Psyschopharmacol Bull.* 1989;25(1):36–40. Medline:2672070

Leonard HL, Swedo SE, Lenane MC, el al. A 2- to 7-year follow-up study of 54 obsessive-compulsive children and adolescents. *Arch Gen Psychiatry*. 1993;50(6):429–439. Medline:8498877

Riddle MA, Hardin MT, King R, Scahill L, Woolston JL. Fluoxetine treatment of children and adolescents with Tourette's and obsessive compulsive disorders: preliminary clinical experience. *J Am Acad Child Adolesc Psychiatry*. 1990;29(1):45–48. Medline:2295577

Riddle MA, Scahill L, King RA, et al. Double-blind, crossover trial of fluoxetine and placebo in children and adolescents with obsessive-compulsive disorder. *J Am Acad Child Adolesc Psychiatry*. 1992;31(6):1062–1069. Medline:1429406

50. Which of the following is a side effect of carbamazepine that commonly diminishes with a temporary reduction in dose?

a. agranulocytosis

b. aplastic anemia

c. lupus erythematous–like syndrome

d. pulmonary hypersensitivity

e. headache

Answer: e

Carbamazepine therapy has many side effects. Rare side effects include agranulocytosis, aplastic anemia, lupus erythematous–like syndrome, and pulmonary hypersensitivity. Some side effects typically diminish with temporary reductions in dose, including ataxia, blurred vision, diplopia, dizziness, fatigue, drowsiness, headache, and nausea.

READINGS AND REFERENCES
Kay J, Tasman A. *Essentials of Psychiatry*. Chichester, UK: John Wiley & Sons; 2006:960.

Multiple-choice exam 3

1. **Which of the following statements is true about buprenorphine?**
   a. It is a full μ-receptor agonist.
   b. It relieves opioid withdrawal symptoms and cravings for 24 hours or more.
   c. Chronic opioid users are likely to abuse buprenorphine.
   d. Buprenorphine can be combined with concurrent behaviour therapies.
   e. Buprenorphine is metabolized primarily in the kidneys.

2. **Which of the following statements about obsessive-compulsive disorder (OCD) and obsessive-compulsive personality disorder (OCPD) is true?**
   a. Obsessions are prominent in both conditions.
   b. In both OCD and OCPD, the impairments are ego-dystonic.
   c. Selective serotonin reuptake inhibitors (SSRIs) are the primary treatment for both conditions.
   d. Anxiety is a prominent component of OCD and OCPD.
   e. Both OCD and OCPD are chronic conditions.

3. Which of the following statements about lithium therapy is not true?
   a. Trials have shown that lithium therapy reduces suicide by 80% in patients with bipolar illness.
   b. Levels above 0.75 mmol/L offer additional protection only against manic symptoms.
   c. The optimal range in patients who have unipolar depression is between 0.6 mmol/L and 0.75 mmol/L.
   d. Lithium reduces glomerular filtration rates (eGFR): eGFR should be checked before prescribing lithium.
   e. Lithium is effective in treating moderate to severe mania, with a number needed to treat (NNT) of 6.

4. Which of the following statements about electroconvulsive therapy (ECT) is true?
   a. It is effective on negative symptoms of schizophrenia.
   b. It decreases positive symptoms of schizophrenia.
   c. It is contraindicated in schizophrenic patients who are pregnant.
   d. Comorbid personality disorders improve after ECT.
   e. Mortality rates for treatment with ECT are higher than for treatment with antidepressant medications.

5. According to current treatment guidelines, which of following is not a condition for which combined pharmacological and psychotherapy may be useful?
   a. psychosocial issues
   b. intrapsychic conflicts
   c. significant interpersonal problems
   d. dysthymia
   e. a co-occurring Axis II disorder

6. Which of the following statements about the effects of cocaine is true?
   a. Cocaine decreases dopamine levels by binding to dopamine receptors.
   b. The blockade of reuptake of serotonin leads to sympathomimetic syndrome, associated with cocaine use.
   c. Metabolites of cocaine can be present in urine for up to 24 hours.
   d. Behavioural effects of cocaine can last up to a day or more.
   e. Repeated administration of cocaine is needed to develop psychological dependence.

7. Which of the following medications may increase plasma levels of methadone?
   a. carbamazepine
   b. phenobarbital
   c. phenytoin
   d. risperidone
   e. fluoxetine

8. Which of the following pairings correctly describe a stage in Erikson's epigenetic model of development?
   a. identity versus inferiority
   b. intimacy versus initiative
   c. autonomy versus guilt
   d. generativity versus stagnation
   e. ego integrity versus isolation

9. Which of the following is not a known risk factor for drug-induced hepatotoxicity?
   a. age
   b. male gender
   c. substance abuse
   d. body weight
   e. genetic predisposition

10. Which of the following phases of Sigmund Freud's model of psychosocial development is paired with the correct age range?
    a. oral phase: 1 to 3 years
    b. shift in libidinal energy to the genitals: 1 to 3 years
    c. phallic phase: 3 to 5 years
    d. latency phase: 11 to 18 years
    e. genital phase: 6 to 10 years

11. Which of the following statements about neurotransmitters and sleep electroencephalograms (EEGs) is true?
    a. Increased rapid eye movement (REM) sleep is associated with adrenergic activity.
    b. Decreased non-REM sleep is associated with serotoninergic activity.
    c. Dopamine is associated with increased REM sleep.
    d. Cholinergic activity is associated with drowsiness.
    e. Adrenergic activity is associated with increased non-REM sleep.

12. Which of the following statements about Gerstmann syndrome is not true?
    a. It is associated with lesions in the nondominant parietal lobe.
    b. Patients can present with right-left disorientation.
    c. Finger agnosia is a typical symptom.
    d. It is associated with dysgraphia.
    e. It is associated with dyscalculia.

13. Which of the following cells is not part of the central nervous system?
    a. astrocytes
    b. Schwann cells
    c. microglia
    d. ependyma
    e. oligodendroglia

14. Which of the following is true about the Hamilton Depression Rating Scale?
    a. It is a clinician-rated instrument.
    b. It is a diagnostic instrument.
    c. It focuses more on biological symptoms of depression.
    d. The interrater reliability of the scale is poor.
    e. The scale has 20 items.

15. Which of the following statements about dementia associated with the human immunodeficiency virus (HIV-associated dementia, or HAD) is true?
    a. Only a minority of HIV patients develops a cognitive disorder.
    b. Aphasia is an early manifestation of HAD.
    c. A mini–mental state exam (MMSE) is a sensitive tool for diagnosing HAD.
    d. Impairment of memory is very prominent in HAD.
    e. HAD is a type of subcortical dementia.

16. Which of the following is a feature of Huntington disease?
    a. It is an autosomal recessive condition.
    b. Increased γ-aminobutyric acid (GABA) levels are seen.
    c. It is associated with a defective trinucleotide repeat of CAG (cytosine-adenine-guanine).
    d. It is associated with decreased dopamine transmission.
    e. It is associated with changes on chromosome 13.

17. Which of the following statements is true about fragile X syndrome (FXS)?
    a. There is a constriction at the end of the short arm of the X chromosome.
    b. It is more common in certain ethnic groups.
    c. It is the most common inherited form of mental retardation.
    d. Many patients with fragile X syndrome have autistic disorders.
    e. There is an unstable DNA sequence of ATT.

18. Which of the following statements is true about autism spectrum disorder (ASD)?
    a. ASD is a global developmental disorder.
    b. The prevalence of ASD approximately 5%.
    c. The symptoms are typically seen after age 3.
    d. It is a degenerative disorder.
    e. It is diagnosed 4 times more often in males than in females.

19. Which of the following statements about persistent depressive disorder (PDD) is true?
    a. Duration of mood disturbance is at least 2 years in children and adolescents.
    b. The 12-month prevalence is approximately 2%.
    c. PDD is associated with an increased risk for subsequent substance-use disorder.
    d. Studies have shown that early onset of PDD is strongly associated with Cluster A personality traits.
    e. For PDD, early onset is defined as before age 18.

20. Which of the following is not characteristic of pediatric autoimmune neuropsychiatric disorders associated with streptococcal infections (PANDAS)?
    a. presence of OCD
    b. prepubertal symptom onset
    c. associated neurological abnormalities
    d. stereotypes
    e. presence of a tic disorder

21. Which of the following statements about the epidemiology of childhood abuse is false?
    a. Studies have shown that boys are at higher risk than girls for fatal maltreatment.
    b. Children born to mothers younger than 21 are at higher risk for childhood abuse.
    c. The most common age of initial sexual abuse is between 8 and 11 years.
    d. Perpetrators of abuse against boys are usually related to the victim.
    e. Boys are less likely to disclose abuse.

22. Which of the following correctly pairs a personality disorder with its common clinical presentation?
    a. borderline personality disorder: pervasive, persistent, and inappropriate mistrust of people
    b. schizotypal personality disorder: emotional detachment and indifference to the world
    c. schizoid personality disorder: cognitive, perceptual, and behavioural eccentricities
    d. paranoid personality disorder: affective instability and rapidly shifting moods
    e. obsessive-compulsive personality disorder: perfectionism and lack of compromise

23. Which of the following techniques is not used in psychoanalysis?
    a. exploration of dreams
    b. examination of symbolism
    c. interpretation
    d. dealing with negative automatic thoughts
    e. free association

24. Which of the following is not a characteristic pathological feature of Alzheimer disease?
    a. neuritic senile plaques
    b. neurofibrillary tangles
    c. β-amyloid protein deposits
    d. granulovacuolar degeneration
    e. lobar atrophy

25. Which of the following is a major risk for dementia?
    a. age
    b. education

c. socioeconomic status
d. occupation
e. obesity

26. Which of the following is not a mechanism of antipsychotic-induced weight gain?
    a. 5-HT$_{2Ac}$ antagonism
    b. hyperprolactinemia
    c. H$_1$ antagonism
    d. serum leptin resistance
    e. low serum iron levels

27. Which of the following statements about the effects of lithium on the cardiovascular and endocrine systems is false?
    a. Benign T-wave changes (flattening or inversion) on electrocardiogram are seen in 55% to 65% of patients.
    b. Bradycardia can result.
    c. Fifteen percent of women report irregular or prolonged menstrual cycles.
    d. Maintenance therapy leads to hyperparathyroidism with hypercalcemia in 10% to 40% of patients.
    e. Clinical hypothyroidism develops in 34% of patients.

28. Which of the following statements about clozapine treatment is true?
    a. Clozapine plasma concentrations are higher in smokers.
    b. Clozapine plasma concentrations are higher in males than females.
    c. The average half-life is 24 to 48 hours.
    d. Agranulocytosis occurs with clozapine in 1 in 1000 patients.
    e. Major motor seizures that occur with clozapine are related to dose.

29. Which of the following is not a risk factor for posttraumatic stress disorder (PTSD)?
    a. female gender
    b. prior mood disorder
    c. family history of anxiety disorder
    d. higher level of education
    e. prior history of trauma

30. Which of the following statements about the hormonal changes associated with aging is true?
    a. Insulin levels are increased.
    b. Thyroxin levels are decreased.
    c. Glucose levels do not change.
    d. Cortisol levels are increased.
    e. Triglycerides are decreased.

31. Which of the following statements is true about the criteria for attenuated psychosis syndrome?
    a. Prodromal symptoms must have been present at least twice per week for the past month.
    b. Prodromal symptoms must have begun in the past month.
    c. Prodromal symptoms could be associated with depression.
    d. Presence of positive symptoms suggests a poor outcome.
    e. The 1-year transition rate to a psychotic disorder is approximately 30%.

32. Which of the following features is not seen in conduct disorder with a specifier of limited prosocial emotions?
    a. lack of guilt
    b. lack of empathy
    c. aggressive outbursts
    d. lack of concern about school or other performance
    e. shallow affect

33. Which of the following neuropsychological tests does not assess memory in geriatric patients?
    a. Selective Reminding Test
    b. Rey Auditory Verbal Learning Test
    c. Wechsler Memory Scale
    d. Wisconsin Card-Sorting Test
    e. California Verbal Learning Test

34. Which of the following statements about Ganser syndrome is true?
    a. Patients give approximate answers.
    b. Patients exhibit clear consciousness.
    c. Patients are oriented in time and place.
    d. Personal information is retained.
    e. Ganser syndrome is more common in women.

35. Which of the following statements about memantine is true?
    a. It is used only in the treatment of severe Alzheimer disease.
    b. It blocks the N-methyl-D-aspartic acid (NMDA) subtype of glutamate receptors.
    c. Elevated transaminases are a known side effect.
    d. Sinus bradycardia is a recognized side effect.
    e. Memantine is contraindicated in patients with hepatic dysfunction.

36. Which of the following statements about body dysmorphic disorder (BDD) is true?
    a. The mean age at disorder onset is older than 20.
    b. The prevalence is much higher in females.
    c. BDD has been associated with high rates of childhood neglect.
    d. Patients are at a lower risk of suicide because they are more concerned with their physical appearance.
    e. There is no association with OCD.

37. Which of the following statements about postpartum psychiatric disorders is true?
    a. The incidence of postpartum psychosis is 1 in 10 000.
    b. Almost 80% of postpartum psychotic patients show symptoms suggestive of schizophreniform disorder.
    c. A history of major depressive disorder increases the risk of postpartum depression.
    d. The Edinburgh Postnatal Depression Scale (EPDS) assesses symptoms of depression in postpartum women within the past month.
    e. The "peripartum onset" specifier in *DSM-5* is applied only for depression with onset during the 12 months after childbirth.

38. Which of the following conditions is not seen in the culture-bound syndrome of latah?
    a. catatonia
    b. echopraxia
    c. echolalia
    d. command obedience
    e. trancelike behaviour

39. You have created a self-rating scale that screens for depression in the indigenous population of a certain geographic area. The findings are as follows:

	DEPRESSION PRESENT	DEPRESSION ABSENT	
Test positive	15	55	70
Test negative	45	125	170
	60	180	

What is the sensitivity of this depression scale?
   a. 0.69
   b. 0.21
   c. 0.96
   d. 0.25
   e. 1

40. Which of the following is a reality distortion symptom of schizophrenia?
   a. delusions
   b. thought form disorder
   c. inappropriate affect
   d. poverty of speech
   e. blunted affect

41. An 80-year-old man, who is currently severely depressed, is taking an SSRI in combination with medications for his physical problems. Which of the following statements is true about his competence to make decisions concerning his treatment?
   a. His competence can only be determined by his psychiatrist.
   b. His competence can be assessed by asking him questions about his financial situation.
   c. He should appreciate all the consequences of his treatment.
   d. His competence involves his ability to understand the information relevant to treatment decisions.
   e. If he becomes floridly psychotic, he will never return to competency.

42. Which of the following is true about kleptomania?
   a. It involves stealing objects needed for personal use.
   b. Affected individuals steal to show anger toward shop owners.
   c. It is a very common condition in men.
   d. There is an increasing sense of tension before the act.
   e. Affected individuals are not aware that their actions are wrong.

43. In an elderly patient, which of the following favours dementia over depression?
    a. rapid onset
    b. short duration of symptoms
    c. complaints from the patient about symptoms
    d. evidence of other cortical dysfunction
    e. no fluctuation in symptoms

44. Which of the following indicators is not annually monitored in patients with chronic schizophrenia?
    a. blood pressure
    b. fasting blood glucose
    c. waist circumference
    d. family history
    e. fasting lipids

45. You are asked to see a 44-year-old male patient, who has had nothing to eat or drink since his admission. He has been sitting for a long period, with minimal interactions with staff. Which of the following clinical features suggests that he has a severe depressive disorder with atypical features?
    a. significant weight loss
    b. excessive guilt
    c. hypersomnia
    d. excessive agitation
    e. worsening of his depression in the morning

46. Which of the following alters with aging?
    a. red cell functioning
    b. bone marrow mass
    c. number of platelets
    d. white cell count
    e. thyroid functioning

47. Which of the following statements about trichotillomania is true?
    a. It is equally prevalent in males and females.
    b. Childhood trichotillomania occurs more in girls than boys.
    c. Late onset is associated with good prognosis.
    d. If it coexists with a psychotic disorder, both conditions can be diagnosed together.
    e. It is more common in individuals with OCD.

48. Which of the following laboratory findings is seen in anorexia nervosa?
    a. hypernatremia
    b. increased liothyronine (T_3)
    c. hypokalemia
    d. metabolic acidosis
    e. leukocytosis

49. Which of the following cognitive functions changes in the elderly?
    a. remote memory
    b. procedural memory
    c. sensory memory
    d. motor speed
    e. executive functioning

50. Structural family therapy highlights the roles of family members within the structure of their families, which opens the possibility of changing the structure to solve problems. Which of the following is not an element of family structure?
    a. coalition
    b. alliance
    c. hierarchy
    d. empathy
    e. boundaries

ANSWERS: MULTIPLE-CHOICE EXAM 3

1. Which of the following statements is true about buprenorphine?
a. It is a full μ-receptor agonist.
b. It relieves opioid withdrawal symptoms and cravings for 24 hours or more.
c. Chronic opioid users are likely to abuse buprenorphine.
d. Buprenorphine can be combined with concurrent behaviour therapies.
e. Buprenorphine is metabolized primarily in the kidneys.

Answer: d

Buprenorphine is a partial μ-receptor agonist; by contrast, methadone is a μ-receptor agonist. With other agents such as methadone and clonidine, buprenorphine is used in the management of opioid withdrawal. It is more effective than clonidine (an α_2-adrenergic agonist) in reducing symptoms of withdrawal.

The advantages of buprenorphine over methadone include:
- lower risk of toxicity at higher doses
- less abuse potential due to partial activation of receptors
- less severe withdrawal symptoms after discontinuation
- more accessible for office-based treatments

Buprenorphine is metabolized primarily in the liver via cytochrome P450. In Canada, physicians do not need special authorization to prescribe buprenorphine, but in some jurisdictions, including the United States, physicians are expected to have a license to prescribe.

READINGS AND REFERENCES
Donaher PA, Welsh C. Managing opioid addiction with buprenorphine. *Am Fam Physician*. 2006;73(9):1573–1578. Medline:16719249
Virani AS, Bezchlibnyk-Butler KZ, Jeffries JJ, Procyshyn RM, eds. *Clinical Handbook of Psychotropic Drugs*. 18th ed. Toronto: Hogrefe Publishing; 2009:292.

2. Which of the following statements about obsessive-compulsive disorder (OCD) and obsessive-compulsive personality disorder (OCPD) is true?
a. Obsessions are prominent in both conditions.
b. In both OCD and OCPD, the impairments are ego-dystonic.
c. Selective serotonin reuptake inhibitors (SSRIs) are the primary treatment for both conditions.
d. Anxiety is a prominent component of OCD and OCPD.
e. Both OCD and OCPD are chronic conditions.

Answer: e

DSM-5 classifies OCD under obsessive-compulsive and related disorders; it classifies OCPD as a Cluster C disorder in personality disorders.

OCD and OCPD differ in several key ways (see the breakdown that follows).

FEATURE	OCD	OCPD
Obsessions, compulsions	Diagnosed by the presence of obsessions or compulsions or both (both obsessions and compulsions are present in approximately 80% of patients)	None
Symptoms	Ego-dystonic	Ego-syntonic
Anxiety	Severe	Not prominent
Treatment	Primarily SSRIs and cognitive behavioural therapy (CBT)	Primarily psychological therapy

The 2 disorders are sometimes, but not often, comorbid.

READINGS AND REFERENCES
American Psychiatric Association. *Diagnostic and Statistical Manual of Mental Disorders.* 5th ed. Washington, DC: American Psychiatric Publishing; 2013:237–242,678–682.

3. Which of the following statements about lithium therapy is not true?
    a. Trials have shown that lithium therapy reduces suicide by 80% in patients with bipolar illness.
    b. Levels above 0.75 mmol/L offer additional protection only against manic symptoms.
    c. The optimal range in patients who have unipolar depression is between 0.6 mmol/L and 0.75 mmol/L.
    d. Lithium reduces glomerular filtration rates (eGFR): eGFR should be checked before prescribing lithium.
    e. Lithium is effective in treating moderate to severe mania, with a number needed to treat (NNT) of 6.

Answer: c

Optimal lithium levels have been defined for manic symptoms (above 0.75 mmol/L), but the range is less clear in patients who have unipolar depression.

Lithium is effective in the treatment of moderate to severe mania, with an NNT of 6. Limitations for its use to treat mania include:
- a typical response time of at least 1 week
- possible increased risk of neurological side effects if combined with antipsychotics

The NNT to prevent relapse into mania is 10 and into depression 14. Lithium also offers some protection against antidepressant-induced hypomania.

A meta-analysis of clinical trials has shown that lithium therapy reduces both completed and attempted suicide rates by 80% in patients with bipolar illness.

READINGS AND REFERENCES

Baldessarini RJ, Tondo L, Davis P, Pompili M, Goodwin FK, Hennen J. Decreased risk of suicides and attempts during long-term lithium treatment: a meta-analytic review. *Bipolar Disord.* 2006;8(5 Pt 2):625–639. Medline:17042835

Crossley NA, Bauer M. Acceleration and augmentation of antidepressants with lithium for depressive disorders: two meta-analyses of randomized, placebo-controlled trials. *J Clin Psychiatry.* 2007;68(6):935–940. Medline:17592920

Morriss R, Benjamin B. Lithium and eGFR: a new routinely available tool for the prevention of chronic kidney disease. *Br J Psychiatry.* 2008;193(2):93–95. doi: 10.1192/bjp.bp.108.051268. Medline:18669987

National Collaborating Centre for Mental Health. *Bipolar Disorder: The Management of Bipolar Disorder in Adults, Children, and Adolescents, in Primary and Secondary Care.* National Clinical Practice Guideline Number 38. Leicester and London, UK: the British Psychological Society and the Royal College of Psychiatrists; 2006.

Severus WE, Kleindienst N, Seemüller F, Frangou S, Möller HJ, Greil W. What is the optimal serum lithium level in the long-term treatment of bipolar disorder--a review? *Bipolar Disord.* 2008;10(2):231–237. doi: 10.1111/j.1399-5618.2007.00475.x. Medline:18271901

Storosum JG, Wohlfarth T, Schene A, Elferink A, van Zwieten BJ, van den Brink W. Magnitude of effect of lithium in short-term efficacy studies of moderate to severe manic episode. *Bipolar Disord.* 2007;9(8):793–798. Medline:18076528

Taylor D, Paton C, Kapur S. *The Maudsley Prescribing Guidelines in Psychiatry.* 11th ed. Chichester, UK: Wiley-Blackwell; 2012:159–168.

Tondo L, Baldessarini RJ, Floris G. Long-term clinical effectiveness of lithium maintenance treatment in types I and II bipolar disorders. *Br J Psychiatry.* 2001;178(suppl 41):S184–S190. Medline:11388960

4. Which of the following statements about electroconvulsive therapy (ECT) is true?

a. It is effective on negative symptoms of schizophrenia.

b. It decreases positive symptoms of schizophrenia.

c. It is contraindicated in schizophrenic patients who are pregnant.

d. Comorbid personality disorders improve after ECT.

e. Mortality rates for treatment with ECT are higher than for treatment with antidepressant medications.

Answer: b

Studies have shown that ECT decreases positive symptoms of schizophrenia, but has no effect on negative symptoms.

There is no absolute medical contraindication to ECT.
Personality disorders do not improve with ECT.
ECT is a safe procedure, with mortality rates lower than for antidepressants.

READINGS AND REFERENCES
Chanpattana W, Chakrabhand ML. Combined ECT and neuroleptic therapy in treatment-refractory schizophrenia: prediction of outcome. *Psychiatry Res.* 2001;105(1):107–115. Medline:11740980

5. According to current treatment guidelines, which of following is not a condition for which combined pharmacological and psychotherapy may be useful?
   a. psychosocial issues
   b. intrapsychic conflicts
   c. significant interpersonal problems
   d. dysthymia
   e. a co-occurring Axis II disorder

Answer: d

The American Psychiatric Association practice guideline for the treatment of patients with major depressive disorder identifies a broad range of conditions for which combined treatment should be considered. These include all of the conditions listed as possible answers for this question, except dysthymia.

READINGS AND REFERENCES
American Psychiatric Association. Practice guideline for the treatment of patients with major depressive disorder. 3rd ed. *Am J Psychiatry.* 2010;167(10 suppl):1–118.
Busch FN, Sandberg LS. Combined treatment of depression. *Psychiatr Clin North Am.* 2012;35(1):165–179. Medline:22370497

6. Which of the following statements about the effects of cocaine is true?
   a. Cocaine decreases dopamine levels by binding to dopamine receptors.
   b. The blockade of reuptake of serotonin leads to sympathomimetic syndrome, associated with cocaine use.
   c. Metabolites of cocaine can be present in urine for up to 24 hours.
   d. Behavioural effects of cocaine can last up to a day or more.
   e. Repeated administration of cocaine is needed to develop psychological dependence.

Answer: e

The behavioural effects of cocaine are short lived: psychological dependence comes from repeated administration.

Cocaine increases dopamine levels by binding to dopamine transporters and inhibiting their activity. Cocaine also affects norepinephrine and serotonin neurons. Cocaine metabolites remain in urine and blood for up to 10 days.

READINGS AND REFERENCES
Galanter M, Kleber HD, eds. *The American Psychiatric Publishing Textbook of Substance Abuse Treatment*. 4th ed. Arlington, VA: American Psychiatric Publishing; 2008.
Sadock BJ, Sadock VA. *Kaplan and Sadock's Synopsis of Psychiatry: Behavioral Sciences/ Clinical Psychiatry*. 10th ed. Philadelphia: Wolters Kluwer/Lippincott Williams & Wilkins; 2007:423.

7. Which of the following medications may increase plasma levels of methadone?
   a. carbamazepine
   b. phenobarbital
   c. phenytoin
   d. risperidone
   e. fluoxetine

Answer: e

Methadone treatment is known to affect the metabolism of other medications, and causes either increases or decreases in plasma levels.

Carbamazepine, phenobarbital, phenytoin, and risperidone may reduce plasma levels of methadone. Fluoxetine and sertraline may increase plasma levels of methadone. Methadone may increase plasma levels of desipramine and amitriptyline.

READINGS AND REFERENCES
Galanter M, Kleber HD, eds. *The American Psychiatric Publishing Textbook of Substance Abuse Treatment*. 4th ed. Arlington, VA: American Psychiatric Publishing; 2008:293.

8. Which of the following pairings correctly describe a stage in Erikson's epigenetic model of development?
   a. identity versus inferiority
   b. intimacy versus initiative
   c. autonomy versus guilt
   d. generativity versus stagnation
   e. ego integrity versus isolation

Answer: d

Erik Erikson developed an epigenetic model of psychosocial development (in contrast to Freud's 5 stages of id development). Erikson's model has 8 stages as follows:
- basic trust versus mistrust: 0 to 12 months
- autonomy versus shame and doubt: 1 to 3 years
- initiative versus guilt: 3 to 5 years
- industry versus inferiority: 6 to 10 years
- identity versus role confusion: 11 to 20 years
- intimacy versus isolation: 20 to 40 years
- generativity versus stagnation: 40 to 65 years
- ego integrity versus despair: 65 years and older

READINGS AND REFERENCES
Erickson E. *Childhood and Society*. 2nd ed. New York: W.W. Norton; 1963.
Ferrando SJ, ed. *Psychiatry In-Review*. 3rd ed. New York: Educational Testing and Assessment Systems (ETAS); 2008:3.
Sadock BJ, Sadock VA. *Kaplan and Sadock's Synopsis of Psychiatry: Behavioral Sciences/Clinical Psychiatry*. 10th ed. Philadelphia: Wolters Kluwer/Lippincott Williams & Wilkins; 2007:207–213.

9. Which of the following is not a known risk factor for drug-induced hepatotoxicity?
   a. age
   b. male gender
   c. substance abuse
   d. body weight
   e. genetic predisposition

Answer: b

According to Grattagliano et al., the following are known risk factors for drug-induced hepatotoxicity:
- increasing age
- female gender
- alcohol consumption
- coprescription of enzyme-inducing drugs
- genetic predisposition
- obesity
- preexisting liver disease

Drug-induced hepatotoxicity can be due to:
- direct dose-related hepatotoxicity (type I adverse drug reaction)
- hypersensitivity reactions (type II adverse drug reaction), which can present with rash, fever, and eosinophilia

Almost all drugs have been associated with cases of hepatotoxicity, but frequency varies.

READINGS AND REFERENCES

Grattagliano I, Bonfrate L, Diogo CV, et al. Biochemical mechanisms in drug-induced liver injury: certainties and doubts. *World J Gastroenterol*. 2009;15(39):4865–4876. Medline:19842215

Taylor D, Paton C, Kapur S. *The Maudsley Prescribing Guidelines in Psychiatry*. 11th ed. Chichester, UK: Wiley-Blackwell; 2012:485.

10. Which of the following phases of Sigmund Freud's model of psychosocial development is paired with the correct age range?

a. oral phase: 1 to 3 years

b. shift in libidinal energy to the genitals: 1 to 3 years

c. phallic phase: 3 to 5 years

d. latency phase: 11 to 18 years

e. genital phase: 6 to 10 years

Answer: c

Sigmund Freud's stages of psychosexual development are as follows:
- oral phase (0 to 12 months): primary means of gratification is sucking and feeding
- anal phase (1 to 3 years): libidinal energy is focused on bowel habits
- phallic phase (3 to 5 years): libidinal energy is focused on genitals; the Oedipus complex becomes important
- latency phase (6 to 10 years): libido is repressed for pursuit of same-sex friendships, school, and sports
- genital phase (11 to 18 years): libidinal energy is refocused on genitals; sexual peer relationships become important

READINGS AND REFERENCES

Chrzanowski DT, Gold J. Childhood and adolescent development. In: Ferrando SJ, ed. *Psychiatry In-Review*. 3rd ed. New York: Educational Testing and Assessment Systems (ETAS); 2008:4.

Freud, S. *On Sexuality*. London, UK: Penguin Books; 1956.

11. **Which of the following statements about neurotransmitters and sleep electroencephalograms (EEGs) is true?**
    a. Increased rapid eye movement (REM) sleep is associated with adrenergic activity.
    b. Decreased non-REM sleep is associated with serotoninergic activity.
    c. Dopamine is associated with increased REM sleep.
    d. Cholinergic activity is associated with drowsiness.
    e. Adrenergic activity is associated with increased non-REM sleep.

Answer: c

EEGs correlate the following neurotransmitter changes and sleep states:
- histamine: active wakefulness
- cholinergic: wakefulness, REM sleep
- adrenergic: decreased REM sleep
- serotonergic: increased non-REM sleep
- dopamine: increased REM sleep

READINGS AND REFERENCES
Buckley P, Prewette D, Bird J, Harrison G. *Examination Notes in Psychiatry*. 4th ed. London: Hodder Arnold; 2005:185–194.

12. **Which of the following statements about Gerstmann syndrome is not true?**
    a. It is associated with lesions in the nondominant parietal lobe.
    b. Patients can present with right-left disorientation.
    c. Finger agnosia is a typical symptom.
    d. It is associated with dysgraphia.
    e. It is associated with dyscalculia.

Answer: a

Gerstmann syndrome is associated with lesions in the dominant hemisphere, including the angular and supramarginal gyri near the temporal and posterior parietal lobe junction.
 The other answers listed in this question are true.

READINGS AND REFERENCES
Whyte EM, Lombard LA. Organic illness in psychiatry. In: Kupfer DJ, Horner MS, Brent DA, et al, eds. *Oxford American Handbook of Psychiatry*. Oxford: Oxford University Press; 2008:158.

13. **Which of the following cells is not part of the central nervous system?**
    a. astrocytes
    b. Schwann cells

c. microglia
   d. ependyma
   e. oligodendroglia

Answer: b

Schwann cells are part of the peripheral nervous system.
 The other cells listed in this question are the major cells of the central nervous system.

READINGS AND REFERENCES
Puri BK, Hall AD. *Revision Notes in Psychiatry*. 2nd ed. London: Arnold; 2004:173.

14. Which of the following is true about the Hamilton Depression Rating Scale?
   a. It is a clinician-rated instrument.
   b. It is a diagnostic instrument.
   c. It focuses more on biological symptoms of depression.
   d. The interrater reliability of the scale is poor.
   e. The scale has 20 items.

Answer: b

The Hamilton Depression Rating Scale (HAM-D) is a clinician-rated tool with 17 items. It assesses symptoms in the last 7 days and has a score range of 0 to 50. The scoring for depression breaks down as follows:

- < 7: normal
- 8 to 13: mild
- 14 to 18: moderate
- 19 to 22: severe
- \> 23: very severe

The commonly used version of this scale does not assess symptoms of depression such as increased sleep, increased appetite, and psychomotor retardation (biological symptoms).

Psychometric properties for the overall Hamilton Depression Rating Scale—such as internal, interrater, and retest reliability—are mostly good.

READINGS AND REFERENCES
Bagby RM, Ryder AG, Schuller DR, Marshall MB. The Hamilton Depression Rating Scale: has the gold standard become a lead weight? *Am J Psychiatry*. 2004;161(12):2163–2177. doi:10.1176/appi.ajp.161.12.2163. Medline:15569884

Hamilton M. A rating scale for depression. *J Neurol Neurosurg Psychiatry*. February 1960;23:56–62. doi:10.1136/jnnp.23.1.56 PMID 14399272. Medline:14399272

Hedlund JL, Viewig BW. The Hamilton rating scale for depression: a comprehensive review. *J Operational Psychiatry*. 1979;10(2):149–165.

15. Which of the following statements about dementia associated with the human immunodeficiency virus (HIV-associated dementia, or HAD) is true?

a. Only a minority of HIV patients develops a cognitive disorder.
b. Aphasia is an early manifestation of HAD.
c. A mini–mental state exam (MMSE) is a sensitive tool for diagnosing HAD.
d. Impairment of memory is very prominent in HAD.
e. HAD is a type of subcortical dementia.

Answer: e

HAD is a progressive subcortical dementia.

Seventy percent to 80% of HIV patients develop a cognitive disorder and approximately 30% develop HAD.

An MMSE is not sensitive in this situation, but tools such as the HIV Dementia Scale are useful for assessing the severity of cognitive changes.

HAD is slow in onset, and of mild to moderate severity. It presents with affective, behavioural, cognitive, and motor symptoms and signs. Psychomotor slowing is prominent in HAD; impairment of memory and language is less prominent. Note that aphasia, agnosia, and apraxia are late-occurring symptoms in HAD.

READINGS AND REFERENCES
Stern TA, Herman JB, eds. *Massachusetts General Hospital Psychiatry Update and Board Preparation.* 2nd ed. Columbus, OH: McGraw-Hill Professional; 2003:210–211.

16. Which of the following is a feature of Huntington disease?

a. It is an autosomal recessive condition.
b. Increased γ-aminobutyric acid (GABA) levels are seen.
c. It is associated with a defective trinucleotide repeat of CAG (cytosine-adenine-guanine).
d. It is associated with decreased dopamine transmission.
e. It is associated with changes on chromosome 13.

Answer: c

Huntington disease is an autosomal dominant condition characterized by a combination of slowly progressive dementia, chorea, and psychiatric symptoms. The Huntington gene is a fully penetrant gene, located on the short arm of chromosome 4. The genetic defect is in the number of the trinucleotide repeat (CAG), as well as some other changes (e.g., greatly decreased GABA neurons in the basal ganglia). Repeats of more than 35 CAGs are associated with the disease. The more repeats (beyond 35), the earlier the onset of the disease. The disease becomes manifest at earlier ages in successive generations, because repeats tend to increase in length.

READINGS AND REFERENCES
Sadock BJ, Sadock VA. *Kaplan and Sadock's Synopsis of Psychiatry: Behavioral Sciences/Clinical Psychiatry*. 10th ed. Philadelphia: Wolters Kluwer/Lippincott Williams & Wilkins; 2007:333.

Whyte EM, Lombard LA. Organic illness in psychiatry. In: Kupfer DJ, Horner MS, Brent DA, et al, eds. *Oxford American Handbook of Psychiatry*. Oxford: Oxford University Press; 2008:200.

17. Which of the following statements is true about fragile X syndrome (FXS)?
   a. There is a constriction at the end of the short arm of the X chromosome.
   b. It is more common in certain ethnic groups.
   c. It is the most common inherited form of mental retardation.
   d. Many patients with fragile X syndrome have autistic disorders.
   e. There is an unstable DNA sequence of ATT.

Answer: c

FXS is the most common inherited form of mental retardation. It is an X-linked disorder with a very unusual pattern of inheritance. A fragile site on the long (q) arm of the X chromosome at Xq27.3, and the "fragility" of the X chromosome, is now known to be associated with an unstable region of DNA within the fragile X mental retardation 1 (FMR1) gene. The instability is caused by an increase in CGG (cytosine-guanine-guanine) repeats as follows:

- 50 or so repeats: usual
- 50 to 100 repeats: premutation
- more than 230 repeats: full mutation

FXS has a prevalence of about 0.3 in 1000, and it affects all ethnic groups equally.

The clinical presentation in males includes mental retardation, language impairment, gaze aversion, self-stimulatory behaviours, and hyperactivity. Persons with FXS seem to have relatively strong communication skills; however, other common features include social impairment, social anxiety, and avoidance of eye-to-eye contact.

Men with FXS are usually affectionate—a significant difference to autism. Self-injury is relatively common, especially hand biting.

READINGS AND REFERENCES
Clarke DM, Deb S. Syndromes causing intellectual disability. In: Gelder MG, Andreasen MD, López-Ibor JJ Jr, Geddes R, eds. *New Oxford Textbook of Psychiatry*. Vol 2. 2nd ed. Oxford: Oxford University Press; 2012:1839–1840.

Pozdnyakova I, Regan L. New insights into Fragile X syndrome: relating genotype to phenotype at the molecular level. *FEBS J*. 2005:272(3):872–878. Medline:15670167

18. Which of the following statements is true about autism spectrum disorder (ASD)?

a. ASD is a global developmental disorder.
b. The prevalence of ASD approximately 5%.
c. The symptoms are typically seen after the age of 3.
d. It is a degenerative disorder.
e. It is diagnosed 4 times more often in males than in females.

Answer: e

The classification ASD includes only 2 domains:

- persistent deficits in social communication and social interaction across multiple contexts
- restricted, repetitive patterns of behaviour, interests, or activities

ASD is a very specific behavioural condition, and not a global developmental or degenerative disorder.

Its reported prevalence (US and other countries) is 1% of the population (child and adult samples).

Symptoms are usually recognized during the second year of life, but if the condition is severe, symptoms may emerge in the first year.

READINGS AND REFERENCES
American Psychiatric Association. *Diagnostic and Statistical Manual of Mental Disorders.* 5th ed. Washington, DC: American Psychiatric Publishing; 2013:50–59.

19. Which of the following statements about persistent depressive disorder (PDD) is true?

a. Duration of mood disturbance is at least 2 years in children and adolescents.
b. The 12-month prevalence is approximately 2%.
c. PDD is associated with an increased risk for subsequent substance-use disorder.
d. Studies have shown that early onset of PDD is strongly associated with Cluster A personality traits.
e. For PDD, early onset is defined as before age 18.

Answer: c

A detailed description of PDD (dysthymia) can be found in the diagnostic criteria of *DSM-5*. The important features include:

- a persistent depressed or irritable mood that is:
  - present for most of the day
  - present for more days than not
  - present for at least 1 year (in adults, for at least 2 years)

The 12-month prevalence is approximately 0.5% for PDD.

PDD is associated with increased risk for subsequent major depressive disorder (76%), bipolar disorder (13%), and substance abuse (15%).

PDD is strongly associated Cluster B and C personality traits.

Early onset is defined as before age 21.

READINGS AND REFERENCES

American Psychiatric Association. *Diagnostic and Statistical Manual of Mental Disorders.* 5th ed. Washington, DC: American Psychiatric Publishing; 2013:168–171.

Kovacs M, Akiskal HS, Gatsonis C, Parrone PL. Childhood-onset dysthymic disorder: clinical features and prospective naturalistic outcome. *Arch Gen Psychiatry.* 1994;51(5):365–374. Medline:8179460

Kovacs M, Feinberg TL, Crouse-Novak MA, et al. Depressive disorders in childhood, I: a longitudinal prospective study of characteristics and recovery. *Arch Gen Psychiatry.* 1984;41(3):229–237. Medline:6367688

Kovacs M, Feinberg TL, Crouse-Novak M, et al. Depressive disorders in childhood, II: a longitudinal study of the risk for a subsequent major depression. *Arch Gen Psychiatr.* 1984;41(7):643–649. Medline:6732424

Lewinsohn PM, Rohde P, Seeley JR, Hops H. Comorbidity of unipolar depression, I: major depression with dysthymia. *J Abnorm Psychol.* 1991;100(2):205–213. Medline:2040772

20. **Which of the following is not characteristic of pediatric autoimmune neuropsychiatric disorders associated with streptococcal infections (PANDAS)?**

   a. presence of OCD
   b. prepubertal symptom onset
   c. associated neurological abnormalities
   d. stereotypes
   e. presence of a tic disorder

Answer: d

PANDAS are defined by 5 clinical characteristics:

- presence of OCD or a tic disorder (or both)
- onset between age 3 and puberty
- symptoms with dramatic onset, acute exacerbations, and episodic severity
- symptom exacerbations timed with group A β-hemolytic *Streptococcus* infection (GABHS)
- associated neurological abnormalities

READINGS AND REFERENCES

Freeman JB, Garcia AM, Swedo SE, et al. Obsessive-compulsive disorder. In: In: Dulcan M, Wiener J, eds. *Essentials of Child and Adolescent Psychiatry.* Arlington, VA: American Psychiatric Publishing; 2006:441–453.

Swedo SE. Sydenham's chorea: a model for childhood autoimmune neuropsychiatric disorders. *JAMA*. 1994;272(22):1788–1791. Medline:7661914

21. Which of the following statements about the epidemiology of childhood abuse is false?
   a. Studies have shown that boys are at higher risk than girls for fatal maltreatment.
   b. Children born to mothers younger than 21 are at higher risk for childhood abuse.
   c. The most common age of initial sexual abuse is between 8 and 11 years.
   d. Perpetrators of abuse against boys are usually related to the victim.
   e. Boys are less likely to disclose abuse.

Answer: d

The perpetrators of abuse against boys are usually unrelated to the victim.

Other data on the epidemiology of physical and sexual abuse of children includes:

- Male parents or parent figures are the main perpetrators.
- Almost 60% of all victims experience neglect, while 21.3% experience physical abuse, and 11.3% are sexually abused.
- Men were more likely to have experienced physical abuse as a child.
- Psychological and behavioural effects of abuse were more detrimental in female victims.

READINGS AND REFERENCES

Holmes WC, Slap GB. Sexual abuse of boys: definition, prevalence, correlates, sequelae, and management. *JAMA*. 1998;280(21):1855–1862. Medline:9846781

Joshi PT. Physical and Sexual Abuse of Children. In: Dulcan M, Wiener J, eds. *Essentials of Child and Adolescent Psychiatry*. Arlington, VA: American Psychiatric Publishing; 2006:595–613.

Keenan HT, Runyan DK, Marshall SW, et al. A population-based study of inflicted traumatic brain injury in young children. *JAMA*. 2003;290(5):621–626. Medline:12902365

Kempe CH. Sexual abuse: another hidden pediatric problem—the 1977 C. Anderson Aldrich Lecture. *Pediatrics*. 1978;62(3):382–389. Medline:704212

Muram D. The medical evaluation in cases of child sexual abuse. *J Pediatr Adolesc Gynecol*. 2001;14(2):55–64. Medline:11479101

Thompson MP, Kingree JB, Desai S. Gender differences in long-term health consequences of physical abuse of children: data from a nationally representative survey. *Am J Public Health*. 2004;94(4):599–604. Medline:15054012

US Department of Health and Human Services. Abuse and neglect (section HC 210). In: *Trends in the Well-Being of America's Children and Youth 2001*. Washington, DC: Office of the Assistant Secretary for Planning and Evaluation, US Department of Health and Human Services; 2001:142–143.

Yates A. Sexual abuse of children. In: Wiener JM, ed. *Textbook of Children and Adolescent Psychiatry*. 2nd ed. Washington, DC: American Psychiatric Press; 1997:699–709.

22. **Which of the following correctly pairs a personality disorder with its common clinical presentation?**
    a. borderline personality disorder: pervasive, persistent, and inappropriate mistrust of people
    b. schizotypal personality disorder: emotional detachment and indifference to the world
    c. schizoid personality disorder: cognitive, perceptual, and behavioural eccentricities
    d. paranoid personality disorder: affective instability and rapidly shifting moods
    e. obsessive-compulsive personality disorder: perfectionism and lack of compromise

Answer: e

The following list correctly pairs personality disorders with their core features:
- borderline personality disorder: affective instability, rapidly shifting moods, impulsivity, identity disturbance, and recurrent manipulative suicidal and parasuicidal behaviours
- obsessive-compulsive personality disorder: perfectionism and lack of compromise
- paranoid personality disorder: pervasive, persistent, and inappropriate mistrust of people
- schizoid personality disorder: eccentricity and aloofness, combined with emotional detachment and indifference to the world
- schizotypal personality disorder: cognitive, perceptual, and behavioural eccentricities, combined with social ineptitude and discomfort (these patients prefer to be alone)

READINGS AND REFERENCES
Smallwood P. Personality disorders. In: Stern TA, Herman JB, eds. *Massachusetts General Hospital Psychiatry Update and Board Preparation*. 2nd ed. Columbus, OH: McGraw-Hill Professional; 2003:187–194.

23. **Which of the following techniques is not used in psychoanalysis?**
    a. exploration of dreams
    b. examination of symbolism
    c. interpretation
    d. dealing with negative automatic thoughts
    e. free association

Answer: d

All the techniques listed in this question are used in Freudian psychoanalysis, except dealing with negative automatic thoughts. Dealing with negative automatic thoughts is a technique mainly used in cognitive behavioural therapy (CBT).

Some other psychoanalytic techniques include concentration method and examination of parapraxes. Symbolism, displacement, condensation, projection, and secondary revision are some of the mechanisms used in Freud's dream work theory.

READINGS AND REFERENCES
Sadock BJ, Sadock VA. *Kaplan and Sadock's Comprehensive Textbook of Psychiatry*. 9th ed. Philadelphia: Wolters Kluwer/Lippincott Williams & Wilkins; 2009:788–837.

24. Which of the following is not a characteristic pathological feature of Alzheimer disease?
    a. neuritic senile plaques
    b. neurofibrillary tangles
    c. β-amyloid protein deposits
    d. granulovacuolar degeneration
    e. lobar atrophy

Answer: e

Lobar atrophy is seen in Pick disease, and is usually most pronounced in the frontal and/or temporal poles of the cerebral hemispheres.

All the other answers listed in this question are characteristic pathological features of Alzheimer disease.

READINGS AND REFERENCES
Nagy S, Hubbard P. Neuropathology. In: Jacoby R, Oppenheimer C, Dening T, Thomas A, eds. *Oxford Textbook of Old Age Psychiatry*. Oxford: Oxford University Press; 2008:71,77.

25. Which of the following is a major risk for dementia?
    a. age
    b. education
    c. socioeconomic status
    d. occupation
    e. obesity

Answer: a

Risk factors for dementia and Alzheimer disease include:
- age: this is the major risk factor (most consistent and significant)
- sex: many studies show women are at more risk, but some studies have not replicated this finding
- education: some studies have reported an association with low education and age-specific prevalence (e.g., Zhang et al.)
- body-mass index (BMI): higher BMI is a known risk factor (extensively studied)

No clear association has been found with socioeconomic status or occupation.

READINGS AND REFERENCES

Fratiglioni L, von Strauss E, Qiu C. Epidemiology of the dementias of old age. In: Jacoby R, Oppenheimer C, Dening T, Thomas A, eds. *Oxford Textbook of Old Age Psychiatry*. Oxford: Oxford University Press; 2008:391–400.

Gustafson D. Adiposity indices and dementia. *Lancet Neurol*. 2006;5(8):713–720. Medline:16857578

Zhang MY, Katzman R, Salmon D, et al. The prevalence of dementia and Alzheimer's disease in Shanghai, China: impact of age, gender, and education. *Ann Neurol*. 1990; 27(4):428–437. Medline:2353798

26. **Which of the following is not a mechanism of antipsychotic-induced weight gain?**
   a. $5-HT_{2Ac}$ antagonism
   b. hyperprolactinemia
   c. H_1 antagonism
   d. serum leptin resistance
   e. low serum iron levels

Answer: d

All the above mechanisms are associated with antipsychotic-induced weight gain. There is no evidence that drugs exert any direct metabolic effect. However, weight gain can be associated with increased food intake, genetic tendency, and lack of exercise.

Low serum iron levels are involved in akathisia, along with inhibition of presynaptic D_2 heteroreceptors on noradrenaline nerve terminals and compensatory increase of norepinephrine or serotonin.

READINGS AND REFERENCES

Strassnig M, Rock JE. Therapeutic issues. In: Kupfer DJ, Horner MS, Brent DA, et al, eds. *Oxford American Handbook of Psychiatry*. Oxford: Oxford University Press; 2008:1048,1058.

27. Which of the following statements about the effects of lithium on the cardiovascular and endocrine systems is false?
   a. Benign T-wave changes (flattening or inversion) on electrocardiogram are seen in 55% to 65% of patients.
   b. Bradycardia can result.
   c. Fifteen percent of women report irregular or prolonged menstrual cycles.
   d. Maintenance therapy leads to hyperparathyroidism with hypercalcemia in 10% to 40% of patients.
   e. Clinical hypothyroidism develops in 34% of patients.

Answer: a

At therapeutic doses, lithium causes the following changes on electrocardiogram (ECG) in 20% to 30% of patients:
- benign T-wave changes (flattening or inversion)
- QRS widening

Sinus node dysfunction and arrhythmias occur less frequently, but studies have found sinus node dysfunction in following circumstances:
- lithium and carbamazepine used in combination
- high plasma lithium levels
- elderly patients
- patients taking other medications that can affect conduction

READINGS AND REFERENCES
Virani AS, Bezchlibnyk-Butler KZ, Jeffries JJ, Procyshyn RM, eds. *Clinical Handbook of Psychotropic Drugs*. 19th ed. Cambridge, MA: Hogrefe Publishing; 2012:216.

28. Which of the following statements about clozapine treatment is true?
   a. Clozapine plasma concentrations are higher in smokers.
   b. Clozapine plasma concentrations are higher in males than females.
   c. The average half-life is 24 to 48 hours.
   d. Agranulocytosis occurs with clozapine in 1 in 1000 patients.
   e. Major motor seizures that occur with clozapine are related to dose.

Answer: e

Seizures are an important dose-related side effect of clozapine. They affect:
- ~2% of patients at low doses
- ~6% of patients at doses > 600 mg per day

Other features of clozapine treatment include:
- plasma concentrations: higher in certain groups of patients (Chinese patients, nonsmokers, and females)

- half-life: 6 to 12 hours
- agranulocytosis: peak occurs between 4 and 18 weeks, and then falls off sharply; occurs in slightly less than 1 in 100 patients
- pharmacodynamics: potent α1-adrenoreceptor antagonist with a wide range of side effects (e.g., hypotension—low-dose glucocorticoid treatment may be helpful in patients with severe hypotension)

Other side effects of clozapine include: hypersalivation, exacerbation of obsessive-compulsive symptoms, weight gain, somnolence, tachycardia, hypertension, constipation, myocarditis, and cardiomyopathy.

READINGS AND REFERENCES

Alvir JM, Lieberman JA, Safferman AZ, Schwimmer JL, Schaaf JA. Clozapine-induced agranulocytosis. Incidence and risk factors in the United States. *New Engl J Med.* 1993;329(3):162–167. Medline:8515788

Meltzer HY, Bobo WV. Antipsychotics and anticholinergic drugs. In: Gelder MG, Andreasen MD, López-Ibor JJ Jr, Geddes R, eds. *New Oxford Textbook of Psychiatry.* Vol 2. 2nd ed. Oxford, UK: Oxford University Press:1208–1227.

29. Which of the following is not a risk factor for posttraumatic stress disorder (PTSD)?

a. female gender
b. prior mood disorder
c. family history of anxiety disorder
d. higher level of education
e. prior history of trauma

Answer: d

Lower education level is a risk factor for PTSD.
Other risk factors include:

- a history of prior exposure to trauma or chronic stress, particularly at a young age
- female gender (females are at higher risk due to a particular vulnerability to violent assault)
- prior mood and/or anxiety disorders
- low income
- being divorced or widowed

READINGS AND REFERENCES

Halligan SL, Yehuda R. Risk factors for PTSD. *PTSD Research Quarterly.* 2000;11(3):1–7.

30. Which of the following statements about the hormonal changes associated with aging is true?
    a. Insulin levels are increased.
    b. Thyroxin levels are decreased.
    c. Glucose levels do not change.
    d. Cortisol levels are increased.
    e. Triglycerides are decreased.

Answer: d

Many hormonal changes occur with aging and are associated with some psychopathology. For example:
- Cortisol levels are mildly increased and may contribute to depression.
- Hypertriglyceridemia has been associated with delirium.
- Insulin changes have been associated with Alzheimer disease; some studies suggest the enzyme that degrades insulin also degrades β-amyloid protein.

Thyroxin, luteinizing hormones, and glucagon levels do not change during the aging process.

READINGS AND REFERENCES
Agronin ME, Maletta GJ, eds. *Principles and Practice of Geriatric Psychiatry*. 2nd ed. Philadelphia: Wolters Kluwer/Lippincott Williams & Wilkins. 2011:3–13.

31. Which of the following statements is true about the criteria for attenuated psychosis syndrome?
    a. Prodromal symptoms must have been present at least twice per week for the past month.
    b. Prodromal symptoms must have begun in the past month.
    c. Prodromal symptoms could be associated with depression.
    d. Presence of positive symptoms suggests a poor outcome.
    e. The 1-year transition rate to a psychotic disorder is approximately 30%.

Answer: e

Attenuated psychosis syndrome is included in *DSM-5* under conditions for further study. The proposed criteria for diagnosis include:
- 1 or more of the following symptoms (in attenuated form): delusions, hallucinations, disorganized speech
- at least 1 occurrence of symptoms per week for the past month
- worsening symptoms during the past year, or symptoms beginning in the past year

- symptoms that are not better explained by another mental disorder, including a depressive disorder or a bipolar disorder with psychotic features

Important epidemiological features include:
- onset: mid-to-late adolescence
- transition rate to psychosis in help-seeking individuals: 18% in 1 year, 32% in 3 years
  - Transition to a depressive or bipolar disorder with psychotic disorder is possible.
  - Transition to a schizophrenia spectrum disorder is most common.
- outcome: poor outcome with presence of negative symptoms, cognitive impairment, and poor functioning

READINGS AND REFERENCES
American Psychiatric Association. *Diagnostic and Statistical Manual of Mental Disorders.* 5th ed. Washington, DC: American Psychiatric Publishing; 2013:783–785.

32. Which of the following features is not seen in conduct disorder with a specifier of limited prosocial emotions?
    a. lack of guilt
    b. lack of empathy
    c. aggressive outbursts
    d. lack of concern about school or other performance
    e. shallow affect

Answer: c

According to *DSM-5*, conduct disorder should be specified as "with limited prosocial emotions" if it is associated with all of the features listed in this question, except aggressive outbursts.

READINGS AND REFERENCES
American Psychiatric Association. *Diagnostic and Statistical Manual of Mental Disorders.* 5th ed. Washington, DC: American Psychiatric Publishing; 2013:470–471.

33. Which of the following neuropsychological tests does not assess memory in geriatric patients?
    a. Selective Reminding Test
    b. Rey Auditory Verbal Learning Test
    c. Wechsler Memory Scale
    d. Wisconsin Card-Sorting Test
    e. California Verbal Learning Test

Answer: d

The Wisconsin Card-Sorting Test assesses executive function. Other tests for executive function include the Trail Making Test, Symbol Digit Modalities Test, and Short Category Test.

All the other tests listed in this question assess memory and are commonly used for geriatric patients.

READINGS AND REFERENCES
Blazer DG, Steffens DC, eds. *The American Psychiatric Publishing Textbook of Geriatric Psychiatry*. 4th ed. Arlington, VA: American Psychiatric Publishing; 2009:215.

34. Which of the following statements about Ganser syndrome is true?
a. Patients give approximate answers.
b. Patients exhibit clear consciousness.
c. Patients are oriented in time and place.
d. Personal information is retained.
e. Ganser syndrome is more common in women.

Answer: a

The main features of Ganser syndrome are:
- approximate answers (*Vorbeigehen*)
- clouding of consciousness
- loss of personal information
- impaired reality testing
- visual and auditory hallucinations (half of cases)
- other dissociative symptoms (amnesia, conversion disorders)

It is a very rare condition and associated with recent history of head injury or severe emotional stress.

It is approximately twice as common in men as in women.

READINGS AND REFERENCES
Sadock BJ, Sadock VA. *Kaplan and Sadock's Comprehensive Textbook of Psychiatry*. 9th ed. Philadelphia: Wolters Kluwer/Lippincott Williams & Wilkins; 2009:2021–2022.

35. Which of the following statements about memantine is true?
a. It is used only in the treatment of severe Alzheimer disease.
b. It blocks the *N*-methyl-D-aspartic acid (NMDA) subtype of glutamate receptors.
c. Elevated transaminases are a known side effect.
d. Sinus bradycardia is a recognized side effect.
e. Memantine is contraindicated in patients with hepatic dysfunction.

Answer: b

Memantine is thought to act by blocking the NMDA subtype of glutamate receptors in the brain. Some features of memantine include:
- It is used in the treatment of moderate to severe Alzheimer disease (the first drug approved for this).
- Dosing adjustment may be necessary in renal dysfunction.
- Common side effects are dizziness, confusion, headache, and constipation.

Other Alzheimer drugs and their side effects include:
- tacrine: contraindicated in patients with hepatic dysfunction; liver function tests are recommended every other week during dose titration and every 3 months thereafter; elevated transaminases, nausea and/or vomiting, and diarrhea are known side effects
- donepezil: associated with bradycardia, syncope, dizziness, insomnia, abnormal dreams, and muscle cramps
- galantamine: not recommended in severe renal or hepatic impairment

READINGS AND REFERENCES
Agronin ME, Maletta GJ, eds. *Principles and Practice of Geriatric Psychiatry*. 2nd ed. Philadelphia: Wolters Kluwer/Lippincott Williams & Wilkins. 2011:797–798.
Virani AS, Bezchlibnyk-Butler KZ, Jeffries JJ, Procyshyn RM, eds. *Clinical Handbook of Psychotropic Drugs*. 18th ed. Cambridge, MA: Hogrefe Publishing; 2009:240–243.

36. Which of the following statements about body dysmorphic disorder (BDD) is true?
   a. The mean age at disorder onset is later than 20 years old.
   b. The prevalence is much higher in females.
   c. Body dysmorphic disorder has been associated with high rates of childhood neglect.
   d. Patients are at a lower risk of suicide because they are more concerned with their physical appearance.
   e. There is no association with OCD.

Answer: c

BDD has been associated with high rates of childhood neglect and abuse. Other features of BDD include:
- mean age at disorder onset: 16 to 17 years; two-thirds of individuals have disorder onset before age 18
- point prevalence rates: similar in both sexes (2.5% in females versus 2.2% in males)
- suicide attempts: high
- association with OCD: the prevalence of BDD is elevated in first-degree relatives of individuals with OCD

READINGS AND REFERENCES
American Psychiatric Association. *Diagnostic and Statistical Manual of Mental Disorders*. 5th ed. Washington, DC: American Psychiatric Publishing; 2013:242–247.

37. Which of the following statements about postpartum psychiatric disorders is true?

   a. The incidence of postpartum psychosis is 1 in 10 000.
   b. Almost 80% of postpartum psychotic patients show symptoms suggestive of schizophreniform disorder.
   c. A history of major depressive disorder increases the risk of postpartum depression.
   d. The Edinburgh Postnatal Depression Scale (EPDS) assesses symptoms of depression in postpartum women within the past month.
   e. The "peripartum onset" specifier in *DSM-5* is applied only for depression with onset during the 12 months after childbirth.

Answer: c

In patients with a history of major depression, the risk of postpartum major depression is 24%; depression during pregnancy further increases the likelihood of postpartum depression.

Patients are at higher risk of postpartum episodes with psychotic features if:

- They have a personal or family history of depressive or bipolar episodes.
- They lack social support.
- They are single parents.

The incidence of the most serious postpartum illness—postpartum psychosis—is 1 to 2 in 1000. The most common clinical presentations of postpartum psychosis are:

- prominent affective symptoms (80%)
- schizophreniform disorder (15%)
- acute organic psychosis (5%)

EPDS assesses symptoms within the past 7 days, not the past month.

According to *DSM-5*, the "peripartum onset" specifier applies "if the onset of mood symptoms occurs during pregnancy or in the 4 weeks following delivery."

READINGS AND REFERENCES
American Psychiatric Association. *Diagnostic and Statistical Manual of Mental Disorders*. 5th ed. Washington, DC: American Psychiatric Publishing; 2013:186–187.
Burt V, Stein K. Treatment of women. In: Hales RE, Yudofsky SC, Gabbard GO, eds. *The American Psychiatric Publishing Textbook of Psychiatry*. 5th ed. Arlington, VA: American Psychiatric Publishing; 2008:1489–1528.

38. Which of the following conditions is not seen in the culture-bound syndrome of latah?
    a. catatonia
    b. echopraxia
    c. echolalia
    d. command obedience
    e. trancelike behaviour

Answer: a

All of the conditions listed in this question characterize latah (a term of Malaysian origin—different terms are used across Southeast Asia), except catatonia. In Malaysia, latah is more common in middle-aged women.

In latah, stimulus produces an exaggerated startle response: individuals might drop or throw objects in their hands, and speak obscenities. Women of low socioeconomic status comprise most cases of latah.

READINGS AND REFERENCES
Gaw AC. Cultural issues. In: Hales RE, Yudofsky SC, Gabbard GO, eds. *The American Psychiatric Publishing Textbook of Psychiatry.* 5th ed. Arlington, VA: American Psychiatric Publishing; 2008:1538.
Sadock BJ, Sadock VA. *Kaplan and Sadock's Comprehensive Textbook of Psychiatry.* 9th ed. Philadelphia: Wolters Kluwer/Lippincott Williams & Wilkins; 2009:2524.

39. You have created a self-rating scale that screens for depression in the indigenous population of a certain geographic area. The findings are as follows:

	DEPRESSION PRESENT	DEPRESSION ABSENT	
Test positive	15	55	70
Test negative	45	125	170
	60	180	

What is the sensitivity of this depression scale?
    a. 0.69
    b. 0.21
    c. 0.96
    d. 0.25
    e. 1

Answer: d

The sensitivity of this test is 15/60 (25%). Sensitivity is the number of individuals who correctly test positive, out of all those who truly have the condition. It describes the ability of a test to detect a condition.

The specificity of this test is 125/180 (69%). Specificity is the number of individuals who correctly test negative, out of all those who truly do not have the condition. It describes the ability of a test to exclude those who do not have the condition under investigation.

The positive predictive value of this test is 15/70 (21%). This describes the percentage of patients with a positive test result who actually have the condition.

The negative predictive is 125/170 (74%). This describes percentage of patients who do not have the condition out of all those who test negative.

READINGS AND REFERENCES
Lawrie SM, MacIntosh AM, Rao S. *Critical Appraisal for Psychiatrists*. Edinburgh: Elsevier Churchill Livingstone; 2000.

40. Which of the following is a reality distortion symptom of schizophrenia?
a. delusions
b. thought form disorder
c. inappropriate affect
d. poverty of speech
e. blunted affect

Answer: a

Delusions and hallucinations are reality distortion symptoms of schizophrenia.

Thought form disorder, inappropriate affect, and bizarre behaviours are part of disorganization syndrome.

Poverty of speech, blunted affect, and decreased spontaneous movements are part of psychomotor poverty.

READINGS AND REFERENCES
Liddle PF. Descriptive clinical features of schizophrenia. In: In: Gelder MG, Andreasen MD, López-Ibor JJ Jr, Geddes R, eds. *New Oxford Textbook of Psychiatry*. Vol 1. 2nd ed. Oxford: Oxford University Press; 2012:526–534.

41. An 80-year-old man, who is currently severely depressed, is taking an SSRI in combination with medications for his physical problems. Which of the following statements is true about his competence to make decisions concerning his treatment?
a. His competence can only be determined by his psychiatrist.
b. His competence can be assessed by asking him questions about his financial situation.
c. He should appreciate all the consequences of his treatment.

d. His competence involves his ability to understand the information relevant to treatment decisions.
   e. If he becomes floridly psychotic, he will never return to competency.

Answer: d

Competence is a legal term and can only be determined by a court of law. In medicine, it has a specific legal meaning.

In medical situations, competence is known as "decision-making capacity." It is task specific and can be different for each situation.

According to Applebaum and Grisso, a patient has the capacity to give consent if the patient is:

- able to communicate his or her choices
- able to understand the relevant information
- able to appreciate the situation and its consequences
- able to rationally manipulate the information

READINGS AND REFERENCES
Appelbaum PS, Grisso T. Assessing patients' capacities to consent to treatment. *N Engl J Med.* 1988:319(25):1635–1638. Medline:3200278
Martone CA, McGavin CL, Singh A, Hira-Brar S, Paul R, Strassnig M. Forensic psychiatry—civil law. In: Kupfer DJ, Horner MS, Brent DA, et al, eds. *Oxford American Handbook of Psychiatry.* Oxford: Oxford University Press; 2008:830.

42. Which of the following is true about kleptomania?
   a. It involves stealing objects needed for personal use.
   b. Affected individuals steal to show anger toward shop owners.
   c. It is a very common condition in men.
   d. There is an increasing sense of tension before the act.
   e. Affected individuals are not aware that their actions are wrong.

Answer: d

Kleptomania is grouped under impulse-control and conduct disorders.
   It mainly involves stealing objects not needed for personal use.
   Stealing is not committed to express anger.
   The prevalence of kleptomania is unknown, but studies have shown it is a rare condition (prevalence rate is approximately 0.3% to 0.6%). The female:male ratio is 3:1.
   Affected individuals have insight into their condition and are aware their actions are wrong.

READINGS AND REFERENCES
American Psychiatric Association. *Diagnostic and Statistical Manual of Mental Disorders.* 5th ed. Washington, DC: American Psychiatric Publishing; 2013:478–479.

James, DV. Fraud, deception and thieves. In: Gelder MG, Andreasen MD, López-Ibor Jr. JJ, Geddes R, eds. *New Oxford Textbook of Psychiatry*. Vol 2. 2nd ed. Oxford, UK: Oxford University Press; 2012:1942.

43. In an elderly patient, which of the following favours dementia over depression?
    a. rapid onset
    b. short duration of symptoms
    c. complaints from the patient about symptoms
    d. evidence of other cortical dysfunction
    e. no fluctuation in symptoms

Answer: d

Dementia is characterized by:
- insidious onset
- symptoms of long duration
- fluctuations in mood and behaviour
- evidence of other cortical dysfunction (common)

Typical characteristics of depression include:
- consistent mood (low and depressed)
- "don't know" answers
- complaints from patients about forgetfulness

READINGS AND REFERENCES
Baldwin RC. *Depression in Later Life*. Oxford Psychiatry Library. Oxford, UK: Oxford University Press; 2010.

44. Which of the following indicators is not annually monitored in patients with chronic schizophrenia?
    a. blood pressure
    b. fasting blood glucose
    c. waist circumference
    d. family history
    e. fasting lipids

Answer: e

The Canadian monitoring guidelines for most second-generation antipsychotics recommend a baseline monitoring of: personal and family history; weight (BMI); waist circumference; blood pressure; fasting blood glucose; and fasting lipid profile. Apart from baseline monitoring, fasting lipids should be monitored every 5 years.

READINGS AND REFERENCES
Cohn TA, Sernyak MJ. Metabolic monitoring for patients treated with antipsychotics medications. *Can J Psychiatry*. 2006:51(8):492–501. Medline:16933586

45. You are asked to see a 44-year-old male patient, who has had nothing to eat or drink since his admission. He has been sitting for a long period, with minimal interactions with staff. Which of the following clinical features suggests that he has a severe depressive disorder with atypical features?
   a. significant weight loss
   b. excessive guilt
   c. hypersomnia
   d. excessive agitation
   e. worsening of his depression in the morning

Answer: c

Depressive disorder with atypical features has the following clinical signs:
- hypersomnia
- mood reactivity
- significant weight gain
- heavy feelings in legs or arms
- perceived interpersonal rejection

All the other signs listed as possible answers in this question are seen in melancholic depression.

READINGS AND REFERENCES
American Psychiatric Association. *Diagnostic and Statistical Manual of Mental Disorders*. 5th ed. Washington, DC: American Psychiatric Publishing; 2013:184–186.

46. Which of the following alters with aging?
   a. red cell functioning
   b. bone marrow mass
   c. number of platelets
   d. white cell count
   e. thyroid functioning

Answer: b

Bone marrow mass can decrease with age.
   Aging does not affect production of red cells, white cells, or platelets.
   Aging causes change in the thyroid gland, but there is no corresponding change in thyroid functioning.

READINGS AND REFERENCES
Blazer DG, Steffens DC, eds. *Essentials of Geriatric Psychiatry*. 2nd ed. Arlington, VA: American Psychiatric Publishing; 2012:34.

47. Which of the following statements about trichotillomania is true?
a. It is equally prevalent in males and females.
b. Childhood trichotillomania occurs more in girls than boys.
c. Late onset is associated with good prognosis.
d. If it coexists with a psychotic disorder, both conditions can be diagnosed together.
e. It is more common in individuals with OCD.

Answer: e

In *DSM-5*, trichotillomania is included in obsessive-compulsive and related disorders.
Trichotillomania has the following features:
- a prevalence in the general population (adult, 12-month) of about 1% to 2%
- a higher rate of occurrence in:
    - individuals with OCD and their first-degree relatives
    - females: the female to male ratio is 10:1
    - individuals with intellectual disability
- possible association with psychosis, if the disorder begins in adulthood (note that when it occurs in response to psychosis, trichotillomania is not diagnosed at the same time)

READINGS AND REFERENCES
American Psychiatric Association. *Diagnostic and Statistical Manual of Mental Disorders*. 5th ed. Washington, DC: American Psychiatric Publishing; 2013:251–254.
Sadock BJ, Sadock VA. *Kaplan and Sadock's Synopsis of Psychiatry: Behavioral Sciences/ Clinical Psychiatry*. 10th ed. Philadelphia: Wolters Kluwer/Lippincott Williams & Wilkins;781–783.

48. Which of the following laboratory findings is seen in anorexia nervosa?
a. hypernatremia
b. increased liothyronine (T_3)
c. hypokalemia
d. metabolic acidosis
e. leukocytosis

Answer: c

Anorexia nervosa often leads to hypokalemia with hypochloremic metabolic alkalosis, due to excessive vomiting.

Other findings include leukopenia, lymphocytosis, thrombocytopenia, increased blood urea nitrogen, hyponatremia, normal thyroid stimulating hormone (TSH), normal or reduced thyroxine (T_4), reduced T_3, and increased reverse triiodothyronine (rT_3).

READINGS AND REFERENCES
Marcus MD, Wilson DV. Eating and impulse control disorders. In: Kupfer DJ, Horner MS, Brent DA, et al, eds. *Oxford American Handbook of Psychiatry*. Oxford: Oxford University Press; 2008:455.

49. Which of the following cognitive functions changes in the elderly?
    a. remote memory
    b. procedural memory
    c. sensory memory
    d. motor speed
    e. executive functioning

Answer: d

The elderly have reduced motor speed and reaction time.

In general, they show no change in remote, procedural, or sensory memory (although learning time and retention may be impaired).

Surprisingly, studies have shown that executive functioning may remain intact in the elderly.

READINGS AND REFERENCES
Blazer DG, Steffens DC, eds. *Essentials of Geriatric Psychiatry*. 2nd ed. Arlington, VA: American Psychiatric Publishing; 2012:31.

50. Structural family therapy highlights the roles of family members within the structure of their families, which opens the possibility of changing the structure to solve problems. Which of the following is not an element of family structure?
    a. coalition
    b. alliance
    c. hierarchy
    d. empathy
    e. boundaries

Answer: d

All the answers listed in this question are elements of family structure, except empathy.

Family structure is the internal organization of a family, which affects how, when, and to whom family members relate while carrying out their various functions.

Structural family therapy focuses on family rules and roles that characterize the actions of family members.

READINGS AND REFERENCES
Kay J, Tasman A. *Essentials of Psychiatry*. Chichester, UK: John Wiley & Sons; 2006:887.

Multiple-choice exam 4

1. Which of the following symptoms is associated with opiate withdrawal?
   a. slurred speech
   b. coma
   c. increased appetite
   d. insomnia
   e. increased blood pressure

2. Which of the following statements about methadone is true?
   a. It is a partial μ-receptor antagonist.
   b. It immediately suppresses symptoms of opioid withdrawal.
   c. Patients are at high risk of death from methadone in the first 2 weeks of treatment.
   d. It is a short-acting synthetic opioid.
   e. It has a short plasma half-life.

3. Which of the following neurotransmitter changes does not occur after a course of electroconvulsive therapy (ECT)?
   a. increased glutamate
   b. increased γ-aminobutyric acid (GABA)
   c. decreased serotonin
   d. decreased dopamine concentration in the locus coeruleus and substantia nigra
   e. decreased N-acetylaspartic acid

4. Which of the following statements about the side effects of selective serotonin reuptake inhibitors (SSRIs) is true?
   a. Tachycardia occurs more frequently in patients taking SSRIs.
   b. Hyperprolactinemia is associated with all SSRIs.
   c. SSRIs are not associated with weight gain.
   d. The risk of upper GI bleeding is insignificant with SSRIs.
   e. Clearance of all SSRIs is reduced in patients with liver cirrhosis.

5. Which of the following factors is related to good prognosis for schizophrenic patients?
   a. insidious onset
   b. positive symptoms
   c. enlarged ventricles
   d. onset in adolescence
   e. poor premorbid adjustment

6. Based on Bowlby and Ainsworth's attachment theory, which of the following is not an attachment category identified by the "strange situation"?
   a. secure
   b. anxious/avoidant
   c. protesting/despairing
   d. anxious/resistant
   e. disorganized/disoriented

7. Which of the following statements about teratogenicity and mood stabilizers is true?
   a. The incidence of major malformations from lamotrigine use during pregnancy is not related to dose.
   b. Lithium-induced teratogenicity occurs only during the first 2 to 8 weeks after conception.
   c. Lithium is associated with cardiac malformations.
   d. Craniofacial defects are more common with valproic acid than carbamazepine.
   e. Lithium use during pregnancy is associated with diabetes mellitus.

8. Which of the following statements about normal sleep stages is false?
   a. During stage 1, low-voltage waves are seen.
   b. Sleep spindles are mostly seen in stage 3.
   c. Low-voltage K complexes are seen during stage 2 sleep.

d. During stage 3, high-voltage delta waves begin to appear.
e. Delta waves occupy more than 60% of stage 4.

9. Which of the following features is not suggestive of Klüver-Bucy syndrome?
   a. social agnosia
   b. bilateral damage of basal ganglia
   c. hypermetamorphosis
   d. hyperorality
   e. sexual indiscretions

10. Which of the following statements about the Montgomery-Asberg Depression Rating Scale (MADRS) is true?
    a. It has 20 items.
    b. It includes somatic symptoms of depression.
    c. It can be used for assessing patients who are likely to experience side effects from medication.
    d. Scores higher than 20 indicate severe depression.
    e. Each item yields a score of 0 to 6.

11. Which of the following is a finding of Pick disease?
    a. It is an autosomal dominant condition.
    b. Sudden onset of symptoms is common.
    c. Personal conduct is well preserved until late into the illness.
    d. Loss of insight is not a typical feature.
    e. It is a very common disorder.

12. Which of the following statements about statistical concepts is true?
    a. Sensitivity is the probability that a diagnostic test for a disease is positive in a group of subjects who truly do not have the disease.
    b. Specificity is the probability that a diagnostic test for a disease is negative in a group of subjects who truly have the disease.
    c. The correlation coefficient measures the nonlinear relationship between 2 numerical measurements made on the same set of subjects.
    d. The Spearman rank correlation is a parametric correlation that measures the tendency for 2 measurements to vary together.
    e. If the dependent variable is dichotomous, logistic regression is used.

13. Which of the following factors is associated with increased psychiatric morbidity after head injury?
    a. young age
    b. shorter duration of posttraumatic amnesia
    c. a Glasgow coma scale rating of 15
    d. increased duration of loss of consciousness
    e. no previous history of psychiatric disease

14. Which of the following statements about the diagnostic criteria of intellectual disability is true?
    a. Mild intellectual disability is more likely to be diagnosed in females than males.
    b. Adaptive deficits in social participation, independent living, and communication have their onset after the developmental period.
    c. The prevalence of severe intellectual disability is approximately 20 in 1000.
    d. The most common chromosomal abnormality associated with intellectual disability is fragile X syndrome.
    e. The *DSM-5* definition of intellectual disability relies less on specific intelligence quotient (IQ) scores than on other criteria.

15. Which of the following statements about epidemiological data and childhood mood disorders is false?
    a. Depressive disorders affect 0.3% of preschoolers.
    b. Approximately 1% to 2% of elementary school children suffer from depressive disorder.
    c. In adolescents, the lifetime prevalence rate of major depressive disorder is in the range of 15% to 20%.
    d. The lifetime rate of adolescent major depressive disorder is much higher than adult rates.
    e. The point prevalence rates of dysthymic disorder (persistent depressive disorder) in adolescents range between 1.6% and 8%.

16. Which of the following statements about childhood attention-deficit/hyperactivity disorder (ADHD) is false?
    a. Euphoria is a common clinical feature.
    b. Impulsivity is seen.
    c. Six or more symptoms of inattention and/or hyperactivity and impulsivity should be present.
    d. ADHD can be associated with reduced behavioural inhibition.
    e. Very low birth weight conveys a two- to threefold risk for ADHD.

17. Which of the following statements about enuresis is true?
    a. It is more common in boys between the ages of 4 and 6.
    b. The most common etiology is general developmental delay.
    c. The episodes are usually voluntary.
    d. Pharmacologic agents such as desmopressin are the first-line treatment.
    e. To confirm the diagnosis, the frequency of the behaviour should be at least 2 times per week for at least 3 consecutive months.

18. Which of the following statements about neuroleptic-induced tardive dyskinesia is true?
    a. The risk of developing tardive dyskinesia (TD) on typical antipsychotics is 10% to 15%.
    b. Increased age in males is a known risk factor for TD.
    c. A proposed theory for neuroleptic-induced TD is GABA hypofunction, leading to enhanced dopamine transmission.
    d. Positive symptoms of schizophrenia increase the risk of TD.
    e. Symptoms of TD cannot be suppressed consciously.

19. Which of the following statements about interpersonal psychotherapy (IPT) is true?
    a. It is a time-limited therapy.
    b. It was originally designated for severe, chronic, and difficult-to-treat patients.
    c. Validation is the key technique used.
    d. Confrontation of the illness is used.
    e. It is based on eastern contemplative practice.

20. According to Freud, which of the following is not considered part of dream work?
    a. representability
    b. condensation
    c. sublimation
    d. secondary revision
    e. symbolism

21. Which of the following factors is considered a good prognostic factor in obsessive-compulsive disorder (OCD)?
    a. coexisting major depressive disorder
    b. presence of overvalued ideas
    c. presence of schizotypal personality disorder
    d. episodic symptoms
    e. delusional beliefs

22. Which of the following statements about depersonalization disorder is true?
    a. It is an uncommon disorder.
    b. It is more common in males.
    c. Mean age of onset is usually after 30.
    d. A small number of patients report histories of significant trauma.
    e. During depersonalization experiences, reality testing remains intact.

23. Which of the following is not a possible explanation for an observed association in an epidemiological study?
    a. randomization
    b. chance
    c. bias
    d. reverse causality
    e. confounding

24. Which of the following psychometric tests is used to assess a specific cognitive function in the elderly?
    a. Alzheimer Disease Assessment Scale, Cognitive
    b. Dementia Rating Scale
    c. Clifton Assessment Procedures for the Elderly
    d. Behavioural Dyscontrol Scale
    e. Cognitive Performance Test

25. Which of the following is not a possible protective factor in Alzheimer disease?
    a. anti-inflammatory agents
    b. estrogen
    c. apolipoprotein E4 allele
    d. high level of education
    e. apolipoprotein E2 allele

26. Which of the following is a sign of acute phencyclidine (PCP) intoxication?
    a. hypotension

b. bradycardia
c. pinpoint pupils
d. nystagmus
e. respiratory arrest with a pulse

27. Which of the following statements about hoarding disorder is true?
    a. It is a new disorder included in obsessive-compulsive and related disorders.
    b. Up to 80% of hoarders meet the diagnostic criteria of OCD.
    c. Hoarding disorder is a rare condition.
    d. Hoarding symptoms usually occur in the elderly.
    e. Hoarding behaviour is rarely familial.

28. Which of the following statements about disruptive mood dysregulation disorder (DMDD) is true?
    a. The diagnosis of DMDD should be made before age 6.
    b. DMDD is more common in females than males.
    c. Recurrent temper outbursts occur on average 2 times per week.
    d. Chronic and severe persistent irritability is the core feature of DMDD.
    e. The rates of DMDD among children and adolescents are less than 1%.

29. In the context of developmental pharmacokinetics, which of the following is a physiologic characteristic of children, compared to adults, that affects drug action?
    a. smaller body size
    b. less body water
    c. more fat
    d. more plasma albumin to which drugs can bind
    e. bigger volume of distribution

30. Which of the following food products should be avoided if a patient is taking irreversible monoamine oxidase inhibitors (irreversible MAOIs)?
    a. cottage cheese
    b. strawberries
    c. bananas
    d. pineapple
    e. avocados

31. Which of the following statements about brain-derived neurotrophic factor (BDNF) is true?
   a. It is involved in short-term memory in adults in all phases of bipolar disorder.
   b. Serum BDNF increases with each episode of depression.
   c. BDNF is related to substance-abuse comorbidity.
   d. Lithium treatment decreases BDNF levels.
   e. Carbamazepine decreases BDNF levels.

32. Which of the following statements about receptor occupancy and its effects on antipsychotic mechanisms is true?
   a. Targeting serotonin 5-HT$_{1A}$ receptors improves cognitive function.
   b. Targeting 5-HT$_{2A}$ receptors improves positive symptoms.
   c. Muscarinic receptors are involved in the sedative effects of antipsychotics.
   d. Orthostatic hypotension is due to the effect of α_2-adrenergic receptors.
   e. The 5-HT$_{2A}$ effects of antipsychotics cause weight gain.

33. Which of the following statements about lamotrigine is true?
   a. Lamotrigine is thought to act on calcium-channel blockers.
   b. Lamotrigine is metabolized by the liver to an inactive glucuronide conjugate.
   c. The clearance of lamotrigine is not affected in patients with renal impairment.
   d. The majority of rashes induced by lamotrigine are life threatening.
   e. Lamotrigine is structurally related to other antiepileptic agents such as carbamazepine.

34. Which of the following medications is most effective in the first-line treatment of antipsychotic-induced akathisia?
   a. propranolol
   b. clonazepam
   c. vitamin E
   d. atropine
   e. amantadine

35. Which of the following statements about tardive dyskinesia (TD) is false?
   a. It may be caused by dopaminergic receptor supersensitivity in the basal ganglia.
   b. The most common symptom is perioral movements.

c. GABA hypofunction leading to enhanced dopamine transmission could be a cause.
d. The rate of TD is higher in bipolar patients than in schizophrenic patients.
e. Symptoms of TD cannot be suppressed consciously.

36. Which of the following is seen in moderate to severe intoxication of lithium?
   a. anorexia
   b. ataxia
   c. abdominal pain
   d. dizziness
   e. slurred speech

37. Which of the following is not seen in folie à deux?
   a. marked dependence on the primary person
   b. social isolation
   c. low intelligence
   d. psychosis in both principal and associate (always in folie folie simultanée)
   e. association with delusional disorder

38. Which of the following is not part of cognitive behavioural therapy (CBT) for delusions?
   a. clarifying delusions as beliefs, not facts
   b. empirical testing
   c. developing a rationale for questioning delusions
   d. challenging the evidence for delusions
   e. psychoeducation

39. Which of the following is a risk factor for suicide in schizophrenic patients?
   a. male gender
   b. older age
   c. feeling anxious
   d. social isolation
   e. cannabis use

40. Which of the following statements about type I alcoholism is true?
   a. It is the predominant type of alcoholism in females.
   b. The onset is usually before age 25.
   c. It has a high genetic component.
   d. Parental alcoholism is a risk factor.
   e. Parental antisocial behaviour is a risk factor.

41. Which of the following statements about body dysmorphic disorder (BDD) is true?
    a. Compared to OCD, there is less insight in BDD.
    b. The common comorbid diagnosis in BDD is OCD.
    c. The mean age at disorder onset is usually after 18.
    d. The most common worry of BDD patients is their weight.
    e. Suicidal ideation is uncommon in BDD patients.

42. Which of the following statements about stalking behaviour is false?
    a. Most victims are female.
    b. Same-gender stalking is a common problem.
    c. Psychotic disorders are relatively frequent in the intimacy-seekers group of stalkers.
    d. Research has shown that stalkers are more likely to have OCD.
    e. Substance abuse is associated with violence in stalking situations.

43. Which of the following is a neurobiological factor involved in the etiology of depression?
    a. increased brain volume
    b. increased metabolism in frontal and temporal areas
    c. lack of paid employment
    d. low socioeconomic status
    e. low concentration of 5-hydroxyindoleacetic acid (5-HIAA) in cerebrospinal fluid

44. Which of the following tests cannot be used to assess the memory of a patient with mild cognitive impairment (MCI)?
    a. Wechsler Memory Scale, fourth edition (WMS-IV)
    b. Rey Auditory-Verbal Learning Tool (RAVLT)
    c. California Verbal Learning Test (CVLT)
    d. Hopkins Verbal Learning Test (HVLT-R)
    e. Stroop Color-Word Test

45. Which of the following statements about clonidine is true?
    a. Its presynaptic α_2-adrenergic activity increases the release of norepinephrine.
    b. Diarrhea is a side effect.
    c. It reduces activity levels in ADHD.
    d. Hypertension is a known side effect.
    e. It can be stopped immediately because it has no discontinuation symptoms.

46. Among high-risk psychotic youth, which of the following is a predictive factor for progression into a full-blown psychotic disorder like schizophrenia?
    a. unusual, suspicious, or paranoid thought content
    b. male
    c. good academic performance
    d. intellectual disability
    e. medical illness

47. Which of following is not an etiologic or risk factor for enuresis?
    a. positive family history
    b. decreased vasopressin production during sleep
    c. reduced nocturnal bladder capacity
    d. psychosocial stressor
    e. lowered arousal threshold

48. Which of the following statements about Wernicke dysphasia is true?
    a. The primary deficit is in the mechanism by which words are chosen.
    b. There is no defect in the appreciation of the meaning of words.
    c. The ability to speak is not impaired.
    d. Hearing is impaired.
    e. Paraphasic errors are frequent.

49. Which of the following is a test of perception?
    a. Token Test
    b. Boston Naming Test
    c. Graded Naming Test
    d. Bender-Gestalt Test
    e. California Verbal Learning Test

50. Which of the following is an element of structural family therapy?
    a. psychoeducation
    b. communication training
    c. problem-solving training
    d. examining hierarchy of power
    e. thought diaries

ANSWERS: MULTIPLE-CHOICE EXAM 4

1. Which of the following symptoms is associated with opiate withdrawal?
   a. slurred speech
   b. coma
   c. increased appetite
   d. insomnia
   e. increased blood pressure

Answer: e

It is important to differentiate opiate withdrawal symptoms from opiate intoxication, because opiate intoxication is a life-threatening condition.

The symptoms of opiate withdrawal include: anorexia; anxiety; abdominal cramp; broken sleep; craving; dysphoric mood; fatigue; headache; increased blood pressure and pulse; low-grade fever; irritability; headache; lacrimation or rhinorrhea; mydriasis; nausea; vomiting; yawning; muscle and bone pain; and restlessness.

Withdrawal symptoms can be assessed through tools such as the Subjective Opiate Withdrawal Scale, Objective Opiate Withdrawal Scale, and Clinical Opiate Withdrawal Scale.

The symptoms of opiate intoxication include: apathy; dysphoria; psychomotor agitation or retardation; respiratory depression; impaired judgement; pupillary constriction (or pupillary dilatation due to anoxia from severe overdose); drowsiness; coma; slurred speech; and impaired attention or memory.

READINGS AND REFERENCES
Douaihy A, Stowell KR, Kohene SJ, Salloum IM. Substance abuse disorders. In: Kupfer DJ, Horner MS, Brent DA, et al, eds. *Oxford American Handbook of Psychiatry*. Oxford: Oxford University Press; 2008:650–651.

2. Which of the following statements about methadone is true?
   a. It is a partial μ-receptor antagonist.
   b. It immediately suppresses symptoms of opioid withdrawal.
   c. Patients are at high risk of death from methadone in the first 2 weeks of treatment.
   d. It is a short-acting synthetic opioid.
   e. It has a short plasma half-life.

Answer: c

The initial 2 weeks of methadone treatment have a substantially increased risk of overdose mortality: appropriate assessment, titration of doses, and monitoring is crucial.

Other features of methadone treatment include:
- effective maintenance therapy for heroine dependence
- high dependency potential, low lethal dose (controlled drug)
- pharmacodynamics: long-acting synthetic opioid that acts as a μ-receptor agonist
- half-life: 25 hours (average; increases with repeated dosing)

READINGS AND REFERENCES
Virani AS, Bezchlibnyk-Butler KZ, Jeffries JJ, Procyshyn RM, eds. *Clinical Handbook of Psychotropic Drugs*. 18th ed. Cambridge, MA: Hogrefe Publishing; 2009:287–290.

3. **Which of the following neurotransmitter changes does not occur after a course of electroconvulsive therapy (ECT)?**
   a. increased glutamate
   b. increased γ-aminobutyric acid (GABA)
   c. decreased serotonin
   d. decreased dopamine concentration in the locus coeruleus and substantia nigra
   e. decreased N-acetylaspartic acid

Answer: e

Levels of N-acetylaspartate are increased after ECT.

ECT alters several 5-HT receptor subtypes in the central nervous system (CNS).

- 5-HT_{1A} receptors: repeated ECT treatment sensitizes 5-HT_{1A} receptors in postsynaptic neurons, but does not change 5-HT_{1A} receptors in presynaptic neurons (autoreceptors)
- 5-HT_3 receptors: ECT increases the sensitivity of 5-HT_3 receptors in the hippocampus to 5-HT, which triggers increased release of neurotransmitters
- autoreceptors: ECT decreases autoreceptor function in noradrenergic neurons in the locus coeruleus and in dopaminergic neurons in the substantia nigra, which triggers increased release of noradrenaline and dopamine

READINGS AND REFERENCES
Holtzmann J, Polosan M, Baro P, Bougerol T. ECT: from neuronal plasticity to mechanisms underlying antidepressant medication effect. *Encephale*. 2007; 33(4 pt 1):572–578. Medline:18033145

Ishihara K, Sasa M. Mechanism underlying the therapeutic effects of electroconvulsive therapy (ECT) on depression. *Jpn J Pharmacol*. 1999;80(3):185–189. Medline:10461762

4. **Which of the following statements about the side effects of selective serotonin reuptake inhibitors (SSRIs) is true?**
   a. Tachycardia occurs more frequently in patients taking SSRIs.
   b. Hyperprolactinemia is associated with all SSRIs.
   c. SSRIs are not associated with weight gain.
   d. The risk of upper GI bleeding is insignificant with SSRIs.
   e. Clearance of all SSRIs is reduced in patients with liver cirrhosis.

Answer: e

Antidepressants such as SSRIs and serotonin-norepinephrine reuptake inhibitors (SNRIs) are widely used in the treatment of depression because of their tolerability, ease of dosing, and safety.

Side effects associated with SSRIs include:
- weight gain (more commonly reported with paroxetine)
- upper GI bleeding: 2 to 4 times higher risk, especially if combined with nonsteroidal anti-inflammatory drugs (NSAIDs)
- elevated prolactin, which is reported in up to 22% of women on fluoxetine
- cardiovascular effects: bradycardia (occurs more frequently than tachycardia), dizziness, coronary vasoconstriction; use SSRIs cautiously in patients with angina and ischemic heart disease

READINGS AND REFERENCES
Virani AS, Bezchlibnyk-Butler KZ, Jeffries JJ, Procyshyn RM, eds. *Clinical Handbook of Psychotropic Drugs*. 18th ed. Cambridge, MA: Hogrefe Publishing; 2009:4–6.

5. **Which of the following factors is related to good prognosis for schizophrenic patients?**
   a. insidious onset
   b. positive symptoms
   c. enlarged ventricles
   d. onset in adolescence
   e. poor premorbid adjustment

Answer: b

Positive symptoms are related to good prognosis. All the other factors listed in this question are related to poor prognosis.

Other good prognostic factors in schizophrenia include:
- marked mood disturbance during initial presentation (especially elation)
- family history of affective disorder
- good premorbid social and sexual histories

- living in a developed country

Other poor prognostic factors in schizophrenia include:
- onset in childhood (or adolescence)
- negative symptoms
- cognitive impairment
- family history of schizophrenia

READINGS AND REFERENCES

Sadock BJ, Sadock VA. *Kaplan and Sadock's Synopsis of Psychiatry: Behavioral Sciences/ Clinical Psychiatry*. 10th ed. Philadelphia: Wolters Kluwer/Lippincott Williams & Wilkins; 2007:476.

6. Based on Bowlby and Ainsworth's attachment theory, which of the following is not an attachment category identified by the "strange situation"?
   a. secure
   b. anxious/avoidant
   c. protesting/despairing
   d. anxious/resistant
   e. disorganized/disoriented

Answer: c

John Bowlby and Mary Ainsworth developed key theories about childhood attachment. "Attachment" is the reciprocal bond between infants and their primary caregivers, as defined by Bowlby. The "strange situation" is a standardized way to assess attachment developed by Ainsworth.

Based on the theories of Bowlby and Ainsworth, 4 attachment categories can be identified from the strange situation:
- secure: more than 60% of children fit this category by 2 years of age
- anxious/avoidant: these children become less anxious than expected when separated from their primary caregivers; they may have experienced mild parental neglect or resentment
- anxious/resistant: these children demonstrate little spontaneous exploration or become highly distressed upon separation from their primary caregivers; like anxious/avoidant children, they may have experienced mild parental neglect or resentment
- disorganized/disoriented: these children may have suffered severe neglect or abuse; if abused, they exhibit undirected, inconsolable, and highly ambivalent behaviour

READINGS AND REFERENCES

Bowlby J. *Attachment*. Attachment and Loss. Vol 1. New York: Basic Books; 1969.

Chrzanowski DT, Gold J. Childhood and adolescent development. In: Ferrando SJ, ed. *Psychiatry In-Review.* 3rd ed. New York: Educational Testing and Assessment Systems (ETAS); 2008:1–2.

7. Which of the following statements about teratogenicity and mood stabilizers is true?

a. The incidence of major malformations from lamotrigine use during pregnancy is not related to dose.
b. Lithium-induced teratogenicity occurs only during the first 2 to 8 weeks after conception.
c. Lithium is associated with cardiac malformations.
d. Craniofacial defects are more common with valproic acid than carbamazepine.
e. Lithium use during pregnancy is associated with diabetes mellitus.

Answer: c

The following list describes teratogenicity associated with mood stabilizers:

- lithium (avoid in pregnancy, especially the first trimester)
    - cardiovascular malformation (risk ratio 1.2 to 7.7)
    - greater risk for Ebstein anomaly; following lithium exposure during the first trimester, the risk is between 1 in 2000 (0.05%) and 1 in 1000 (0.1%)
    - perinatal toxicity (hypotonia, cyanosis, neonatal goitre, and nephrogenic diabetes insipidus)
- lamotrigine
    - cleft lip and palate: 5.4% increased risk when total dose is more than 200 mg
- valproic acid
    - neural tube defects (rate: up to 5%)
    - spina bifida (risk: 1% to 2%)
    - craniofacial defects
- carbamazepine
    - craniofacial defects (rate: 11%)
    - spina bifida (risk: up to 1%)

READINGS AND REFERENCES

Virani AS, Bezchlibnyk-Butler KZ, Jeffries JJ, Procyshyn RM, eds. *Clinical Handbook of Psychotropic Drugs.* 18th ed. Cambridge, MA: Hogrefe Publishing; 2009:9,191–202.

8. Which of the following statements about normal sleep stages is false?
   a. During stage 1, low-voltage waves are seen.
   b. Sleep spindles are mostly seen in stage 3.
   c. Low-voltage K complexes are seen during stage 2 sleep.
   d. During stage 3, high-voltage delta waves begin to appear.
   e. Delta waves occupy more than 60% of stage 4.

Answer: b

Sleep spindles—short bursts of 12 to 14 Hz activity—appear in stage 2 sleep.

Normal sleep consists of 4 stages:
- stage 1: non-REM sleep; EEG characterized by slower, low-voltage 5 to 7 Hz theta activity
- stage 2: EEG characterized by further slowing of activity, sleep spindles, and high-voltage K complexes
- stage 3: high-voltage delta waves begin to appear
- stage 4: more than 50% of this stage consists of slow delta activity

READINGS AND REFERENCES
Reite M, Weissberg M, Ruddy J. *Clinical Manual for Evaluation and Treatment of Sleep Disorders.* Arlington, VA: American Psychiatric Press; 2009: 17–44.

9. Which of the following features is not suggestive of Klüver-Bucy syndrome?
   a. social agnosia
   b. bilateral damage of basal ganglia
   c. hypermetamorphosis
   d. hyperorality
   e. sexual indiscretions

Answer: b

Klüver-Bucy syndrome arises from bilateral damage of the amygdala and hippocampus. It produces loss of fear and reaction, excessive and indiscriminate sexual behaviour, hypermetamorphosis (forced attention to environmental stimuli), and hyperorality.

READINGS AND REFERENCES
Hooshmand H, Sepdham T, Vries JK. Klüver-Bucy syndrome: successful treatment with carbamazepine. *JAMA.* 1974;229(13):1782. Medline:4479148
Sadock BJ, Sadock VA. *Kaplan and Sadock's Comprehensive Textbook of Psychiatry.* 9th ed. Philadelphia: Wolters Kluwer/Lippincott Williams & Wilkins; 2009:412.

10. Which of the following statements about the Montgomery-Asberg Depression Rating Scale (MADRS) is true?
   a. It has 20 items.
   b. It includes somatic symptoms of depression.
   c. It can be used for assessing patients who are likely to experience side effects from medication.
   d. Scores higher than 20 indicate severe depression.
   e. Each item yields a score of 0 to 6.

Answer: e

The features of the Montgomery-Asberg Depression Rating Scale include:
- assesses the severity of depressive episodes in patients with mood disorders
- is more sensitive to changes triggered by antidepressants and other forms of treatment
- was designed in 1979
- has 10 items
- score range for each item: 0 to 6
- total score range: 0 to 60
- total score: > 34 indicates severe depression

READINGS AND REFERENCES
Montgomery SA, Asberg M. A new depression scale designed to be sensitive to change. *Br J Psychiatry*. April 1979;134:382–389. Medline:444788
Williams JB, Kobak KA. Development and reliability of a structured interview guide for the Montgomery-Asberg Depression Rating Scale (SIGMA). *Br J Psychiatry*. 2008;192(1):52–58. Medline:18174510

11. Which of the following is a finding of Pick disease?
   a. It is an autosomal dominant condition.
   b. Sudden onset of symptoms is common.
   c. Personal conduct is well preserved until late into the illness.
   d. Loss of insight is not a typical feature.
   e. It is a very common disorder.

Answer: a

Features of Pick disease include:
- autosomal dominant
- rare
- underdiagnosed
- primarily diagnosed clinically

- insidious onset
- gradual progression
- early decline in interpersonal conduct (common)
- presentation: alteration in personality, neglect of personal appearance, loss of social awareness, and impulsiveness

READINGS AND REFERENCES
Nagy S, Hubbard P. Neuropathology. In: Jacoby R, Oppenheimer C, Dening T, Thomas A, eds. *Oxford Textbook of Old Age Psychiatry*. Oxford: Oxford University Press; 2008:77.

12. Which of the following statements about statistical concepts is true?
   a. Sensitivity is the probability that a diagnostic test for a disease is positive in a group of subjects who truly do not have the disease.
   b. Specificity is the probability that a diagnostic test for a disease is negative in a group of subjects who truly have the disease.
   c. The correlation coefficient measures the nonlinear relationship between 2 numerical measurements made on the same set of subjects.
   d. The Spearman rank correlation is a parametric correlation that measures the tendency for 2 measurements to vary together.
   e. If the dependent variable is dichotomous, logistic regression is used.

Answer: e

Sensitivity describes the ability of a test to detect a condition among those who truly have the condition. It is the ability of a test to identify those with the condition.

Specificity describes the ability of a test to show negative for a condition among those who truly do not have the condition. It is the ability of the test to exclude those who do not have the condition.

The correlation coefficient, also called the Pearson product moment correlation, measures the linear relationship between 2 numerical measurements made on the same set of subjects.

The Spearman rank correlation quantifies nonparametric values. It does not assume Gaussian distribution or a linear relationship between variables.

READINGS AND REFERENCES
Dawson B, Trapp RG. *Basic and Clinical Biostatistics*. 4th ed. Columbus, OH: McGraw-Hill Companies; 2004.
Lawrie SM, MacIntosh AM, Rao S. *Critical Appraisal for Psychiatrists*. Edinburgh: Elsevier Churchill Livingstone; 2000.

13. Which of the following factors is associated with increased psychiatric morbidity after head injury?
    a. young age
    b. shorter duration of posttraumatic amnesia
    c. a Glasgow coma scale rating of 15
    d. increased duration of loss of consciousness
    e. no previous history of psychiatric disease

Answer: d

Factors associated with increased psychiatric morbidity following head injury include (among others):

- longer duration of loss of consciousness
- longer duration of posttraumatic amnesia
- older age

A Glasgow coma scale rating of 12 to 15 is suggestive of mild brain injury, which may not be associated with increased psychiatric morbidity.

READINGS AND REFERENCES

Rao V, Lyketsos C. Neuropsychiatric sequelae of traumatic brain injury. *Psychosomatics.* 2000;41(2):95–96. Medline:10749946

Whyte EM, Lombard LA. Organic illness in psychiatry. In: Kupfer DJ, Horner MS, Brent DA, et al, eds. *Oxford American Handbook of Psychiatry.* Oxford: Oxford University Press; 2008:180.

14. Which of the following statements about the diagnostic criteria of intellectual disability is true?
    a. Mild intellectual disability is more likely to be diagnosed in females than males.
    b. Adaptive deficits in social participation, independent living, and communication have their onset after the developmental period.
    c. The prevalence of severe intellectual disability is approximately 20 in 1000.
    d. The most common chromosomal abnormality associated with intellectual disability is fragile X syndrome.
    e. The *DSM-5* definition of intellectual disability relies less on specific IQ scores than on other criteria.

Answer: e

The *DSM-5* definition of intellectual disability relies more on adaptive functioning and less on specific IQ scores.

Males are more likely than females to be diagnosed with both mild and severe forms of intellectual disability (the male:female ratio is 1.2:1).

The onset of intellectual and adaptive deficits begins during the developmental period. Severe deficits usually become apparent within the first 2 years of life.

Overall, the prevalence of intellectual disability is about 1%. Severe intellectual disability affects approximately 6 in 1000.

The most common chromosomal abnormality associated with intellectual disability is Down syndrome.

READINGS AND REFERENCES
American Psychiatric Association. *Diagnostic and Statistical Manual of Mental Disorders.* 5th ed. Washington, DC: American Psychiatric Publishing; 2013:33–40.

15. **Which of the following statements about epidemiological data and childhood mood disorders is false?**
   a. Depressive disorders affect 0.3% of preschoolers.
   b. Approximately 1% to 2% of elementary school children suffer from depressive disorders.
   c. In adolescents, the lifetime prevalence rate of major depressive disorder is in the range of 15% to 20%.
   d. The lifetime rate of adolescent major depressive disorder is much higher than adult rates.
   e. The point prevalence rates of dysthymic disorder (persistent depressive disorder) in adolescents range between 1.6% and 8%.

Answer: d

The lifetime prevalence rate of major depressive disorder in adolescents has been estimated at 15% to 20%, which is *comparable* to the rate in adults.

All the other statements listed as answers to this question are correct.

READINGS AND REFERENCES
Anderson JC, Williams S, McGee R, Silva PA. DSM-III disorders in preadolescent children: prevalence in a large sample from the general population. *Arch Gen Psychiatry.* 1987;44(1):69–76. Medline:2432848

Bird HR, Canino G, Rubio-Stipec M, et al. Estimates of the prevalence of childhood maladjustment in a community survey in Puerto Rico: the use of combined measures. *Arch Gen Psychiatry.* 1988;45(12):1120–1126. Medline:3264147

Kashani JH, Beck NC, Hoeper EW, et al. Psychiatric disorders in a community sample of adolescents. *Am J Psychiatry.* 1987;144(5):584–589. Medline:3495187

Kessler RC, McGonagle KA, Zhao S, et al. Lifetime and 12-month prevalence of DSM-III-R psychiatric disorders in the United States: results from the National Comorbidity Survey. *Arch Gen Psychiatry.* 1994;51(1):8–19. Medline:8279933

Lewinsohn PM, Duncan E, Stanton AK, Hautzinger M. Age at first onset for nonbipolar depression. *J Abnorm Psychol.* 1986;95(4):378–383. Medline:3805502

Lewinsohn PM, Hops H, Roberts RE, Seeley JR, Andrews JA. Adolescent psychopathology: I. Prevalence and incidence of depression and other DSM-III-R disorders in high school students. *J Abnorm Psychol*. 1993;102(1):133–144. Medline:8436689

16. Which of the following statements about childhood attention-deficit/ hyperactivity disorder (ADHD) is false?

a. Euphoria is a common clinical feature.
b. Impulsivity is seen.
c. Six or more symptoms of inattention and/or hyperactivity and impulsivity should be present.
d. ADHD can be associated with reduced behavioural inhibition.
e. Very low birth weight conveys a two- to threefold risk for ADHD.

Answer: a

According to current *DSM-5* criteria, a diagnosis of ADHD requires:
- presence of several (6 or more) symptoms of hyperactive-impulsive symptoms before age 12
- presence of symptoms in 2 or more settings
- association of symptoms with disturbance in the quality of social, academic, or occupational functioning
- symptoms not due other mental disorders

READINGS AND REFERENCES
American Psychiatric Association. *Diagnostic and Statistical Manual of Mental Disorders*. 5th ed. Washington, DC: American Psychiatric Publishing; 2013:59–61.

17. Which of the following statements about enuresis is true?

a. It is more common in boys between the ages of 4 and 6.
b. The most common etiology is general developmental delay.
c. The episodes are usually voluntary.
d. Pharmacologic agents such as desmopressin are the first-line treatment.
e. To confirm the diagnosis, the frequency of the behaviour should be at least 2 times per week for at least 3 consecutive months.

Answer: e

There are 3 subtypes of enuresis: nocturnal only (most common), diurnal only, and nocturnal and diurnal. According to *DSM-5*, a diagnosis of enuresis can be confirmed if the behaviour occurs least 2 times per week for at least 3 consecutive months. (By contrast, *DSM-5* defines encopresis as at least 1 event per month for at least 3 months).

Enuresis is equally common in girls and boys between the ages of 4 and 6. After age 11, boys are twice as likely as girls to be symptomatic.

No single cause of enuresis has been identified, but genetics plays an important role. Seventy-five percent of patients have a family history.

The episodes are involuntary.

Enuresis is mostly a self-limiting condition. Reassurance and support are important for affected children to prevent secondary emotional effects. Simple interventions can be effective (e.g., fluid restriction, encouragement of nighttime urination, pads, and bladder training). Other interventions include enuresis alarms and pharmacological agents (e.g., desmopressin, imipramine).

READINGS AND REFERENCES

American Psychiatric Association. *Diagnostic and Statistical Manual of Mental Disorders.* 5th ed. Washington, DC: American Psychiatric Publishing; 2013:355–357.

Schlesinger AB, Horner MS, Malley E, et al. Child and adolescent psychiatry. In: Kupfer DJ, Horner MS, Brent DA, et al, eds. *Oxford American Handbook of Psychiatry.* Oxford: Oxford University Press; 2008:722–724.

Walsh T, Menvielle E, Khushlani D. Disorders of elimination. In: Dulcan M, Wiener J. *Essentials of Child and Adolescent Psychiatry.* Arlington, VA: American Psychiatric Publishing; 2006:581–591.

18. **Which of the following statements about neuroleptic-induced tardive dyskinesia is true?**

   a. The risk of developing tardive dyskinesia (TD) on typical antipsychotics is 10% to 15%.
   b. Increased age in males is a known risk factor for TD.
   c. A proposed theory for neuroleptic-induced TD is GABA hypofunction, leading to enhanced dopamine transmission.
   d. Positive symptoms of schizophrenia increase the risk of TD.
   e. Symptoms of TD cannot be suppressed consciously.

Answer: c

Margolese et al. have proposed the following 4 mechanisms for neuroleptic-induced tardive dyskinesia:

- prolonged blockade of postsynaptic dopamine receptors
- postsynaptic dopamine hypersensitivity
- damage to striatal GABA interneurons
- damage of striatal cholinergic interneurons

TD occurs in about 24% of chronically treated patients (in high-risk patients, rates may be as high as 70%). The risk of developing TD on typical antipsychotics appears to be 4% to 5% per year for at least the first 4 years.

The following are known risk factors for neuroleptic-induced tardive dyskinesia:
- old age
- female gender
- history of acute extrapyramidal symptoms (EPS)
- chronic use of high-dose antipsychotics
- concomitant anticholinergic treatment
- presence of comorbid mood disorders
- previous head injury
- alcoholism
- negative symptoms of schizophrenia (not positive symptoms)

Symptoms can be suppressed consciously. They also disappear during sleep. Factors that exacerbate symptoms include distraction, stress, and antiparkinsonian agents.

Some patients experience neuroleptic withdrawal-emergent dyskinesia—which has symptoms similar to neuroleptic-induced tardive dyskinesia—after changing the dose or discontinuing an antipsychotic agent. Neuroleptic withdrawal-emergent dyskinesia is a time-limited condition: if dyskinesia persists, TD should be considered.

READINGS AND REFERENCES

American Psychiatric Association. *Diagnostic and Statistical Manual of Mental Disorders.* 5th ed. Washington, DC: American Psychiatric Publishing; 2013:712.

Margolese HC, Chouinard G, Kolivakis TT, Beauclair L, Miller R. Tardive dyskinesia in the era of typical and atypical antipsychotics—Part 1: pathophysiology and mechanisms of induction. *Can J Psychiatry.* 2005;50(9):541–547. Medline:16262110

Strassnig M, Rock JE, Patterson KR, Stowell KR. Therapeutic issues. In: Kupfer DJ, Horner MS, Brent DA, et al, eds. *Oxford American Handbook of Psychiatry.* Oxford: Oxford University Press; 2008:1062–1063.

19. Which of the following statements about interpersonal psychotherapy (IPT) is true?
    a. It is a time-limited therapy.
    b. It was originally designated for severe, chronic, and difficult-to-treat patients.
    c. Validation is the key technique used.
    d. Confrontation of the illness is used.
    e. It is based on eastern contemplative practice.

Answer: a

IPT is a time-limited, manual-based, diagnosis-focused treatment developed by Gerald Klerman and Myrna Weissman.

It is a well-established treatment for:
- acute and chronic major depressive disorder (MDD)
- acute bulimia nervosa
- bipolar disorder (as an adjunct treatment)

IPT approaches illness—regardless of its etiology—as something it can modify. The common interpersonal issues explored in IPT are:
- role transition
- role disputes
- interpersonal deficits
- grief

All of the other methods listed in this question are used in dialectical behaviour therapy.

READINGS AND REFERENCES
Blanco C, Markowitz j, Weissman MM. Interpersonal psychotherapy for depression and other conditions. In: Gelder MG, Andreasen MD, López-Ibor JJ Jr, Geddes R, eds. *New Oxford Textbook of Psychiatry*. Vol 2. 2nd ed. Oxford: Oxford University Press; 2012:1318–1323.

20. According to Freud, which of the following is not considered part of dream work?
   a. representability
   b. condensation
   c. sublimation
   d. secondary revision
   e. symbolism

Answer: c

The interpretation of dreams by Freud was a landmark study of his own dreams and his patients' dreams. The theory of dream work includes the following mechanisms: symbolism, displacement, condensation, projections, and secondary revisions.

Sublimation is a mature defence mechanism that provides optimal adaptation in the handling of stressors. Other mature defence mechanisms are anticipation, self-assertion, affiliation, altruism, humour, and suppression.

READINGS AND REFERENCES
Sadock BJ, Sadock VA. *Kaplan and Sadock's Comprehensive Psychiatry*. 9th ed. Philadelphia: Wolters Kluwer/Lippincott Williams & Wilkins; 2007:703,798.

21. Which of the following factors is considered a good prognostic factor in obsessive-compulsive disorder (OCD)?

a. coexisting major depressive disorder
b. presence of overvalued ideas
c. presence of schizotypal personality disorder
d. episodic symptoms
e. delusional beliefs

Answer: d

Good prognostic factors in OCD include:
- episodic symptoms
- good social and occupational adjustment
- presence of a precipitating event

The other factors listed in this answer correlate with poor prognosis. Other poor prognostic factors include:
- yielding to (rather than resisting) compulsions
- pediatric onset
- bizarre compulsions
- need for hospitalization

READINGS AND REFERENCES
Sadock BJ, Sadock VA. *Kaplan and Sadock's Synopsis of Psychiatry: Behavioral Sciences/Clinical Psychiatry.* 10th ed. Philadelphia: Wolters Kluwer/Lippincott Williams & Wilkins; 2007:610–611.

22. Which of the following statements about depersonalization disorder is true?

a. It is an uncommon disorder.
b. It is more common in males.
c. Mean age of onset is usually after 30.
d. A small number of patients report histories of significant trauma.
e. During depersonalization experiences, reality testing remains intact.

Answer: e

DSM-5 identifies the essential features of depersonalization as the presence of a persistent or recurrent feeling of detachment or estrangement from one's self. Certain clinical features are common, including: a sense of bodily change; duality of self as observer and actor; and feeling cut off from others and cut off from one's own emotions. During depersonalization, reality testing remains intact.

Depersonalization disorder is a common clinical condition. It is the third most commonly reported psychiatric condition after depression and anxiety.

The male:female ratio for the disorder is 1:1 and the lifetime prevalence is approximately 2%.

The mean age of onset is 16, although the disorder can start in early or middle childhood. If onset is after age 40, an underlying medical disorder should be suspected (e.g., brain lesions or seizure disorders).

Significant trauma—particularly emotional abuse and neglect—has been strongly associated with the disorder. Other etiological factors include: physical abuse; witnessing domestic violence; and unexpected death or suicide of a close family member.

READINGS AND REFERENCES
American Psychiatric Association. *Diagnostic and Statistical Manual of Mental Disorders.* 5th ed. Washington, DC: American Psychiatric Publishing; 2013:302–306.
Sadock BJ, Sadock VA. *Kaplan and Sadock's Synopsis of Psychiatry: Behavioral Sciences/ Clinical Psychiatry.* 10th ed. Philadelphia: Wolters Kluwer/Lippincott Williams & Wilkins; 2007:668–670.

23. Which of the following is not a possible explanation for an observed association in an epidemiological study?
    a. randomization
    b. chance
    c. bias
    d. reverse causality
    e. confounding

Answer: a

Randomization is a process used in randomized control studies.

In epidemiological studies, associations between exposure and disease can be explained by alternative interpretations including chance, bias, reverse causality, and confounding.

READINGS AND REFERENCES
Prince M. Epidemiology. In: Jacoby R, Oppenheimer C, Dening T, Thomas A, eds. *Oxford Textbook of Old Age Psychiatry.* Oxford: Oxford University Press; 2008:51–65.

24. Which of the following psychometric tests is used to assess a specific cognitive function in the elderly?
    a. Alzheimer Disease Assessment Scale, Cognitive
    b. Dementia Rating Scale
    c. Clifton Assessment Procedures for the Elderly
    d. Behavioural Dyscontrol Scale
    e. Cognitive Performance Test

Answer: d

Several psychometric tools are used in assessing cognitive performance in the elderly. Some tools, including the Behavioural Dyscontrol Scale, are used to screen specific cognitive functions.

The Behavioural Dyscontrol Scale measures executive abilities. It was initially designed to predict functional independence in geriatric populations.

The Alzheimer Disease Assessment Scale, Cognitive (ADAS-cog) is commonly used to assess cognitive dysfunction in individuals with Alzheimer disease and other dementias.

The Dementia Rating Scale is a numeric scale that quantifies the severity of dementia symptoms and is used in the differential diagnosis of dementia.

The Clifton Assessment Procedures for the Elderly evaluate mental and behavioural impairments. The procedures comprise a cognitive assessment scale and a behaviour rating scale.

The Cognitive Performance Test is a standardized, performance-based test originally designed for the objective evaluation of cognitive function in Alzheimer disease.

READINGS AND REFERENCES
Ritchie, K. Psychometry in older persons. In: Jacoby R, Oppenheimer C, Dening T, Thomas A, eds. *Oxford Textbook of Old Age Psychiatry*. Oxford: Oxford University Press; 2008:119–128.

25. Which of the following is **not** a possible protective factor in Alzheimer disease?
    a. anti-inflammatory agents
    b. estrogen
    c. apolipoprotein E4 allele
    d. high level of education
    e. apolipoprotein E2 allele

Answer: c

The apolipoprotein E4 allele is a well-established risk factor in Alzheimer disease. Other well-known risk factors include age, family history, and Down syndrome.

READINGS AND REFERENCES
Thomas A. Clinical aspects of dementia: Alzheimer's disease. In: Jacoby R, Oppenheimer C, Dening T, Thomas A, eds. *Oxford Textbook of Old Age Psychiatry*. Oxford: Oxford University Press; 2008:432–435.

26. Which of the following is a sign of acute phencyclidine (PCP) intoxication?
   a. hypotension
   b. bradycardia
   c. pinpoint pupils
   d. nystagmus
   e. respiratory arrest with a pulse

Answer: d

Nystagmus is a sign of PCP intoxication. The other answers listed in this question are signs of opioid overdose.

Other known signs of PCP intoxication include agitation, belligerence, impaired judgement, hyperacusis, hypertension, tachycardia, numbness, ataxia, dysarthria, rigidity, salivation, seizure, and coma.

READINGS AND REFERENCES
Abraham HD. Disorders relating to the use of phencyclidine and hallucinogens. In: Gelder MG, Andreasen MD, López-Ibor JJ Jr, Geddes R, eds. *New Oxford Textbook of Psychiatry.* Vol 1. 2nd ed. Oxford, UK: Oxford University Press; 2012:486–490.

27. Which of the following statements about hoarding disorder is true?
   a. It is a new disorder included in obsessive-compulsive and related disorders.
   b. Up to 80% of hoarders meet the diagnostic criteria of OCD.
   c. Hoarding disorder is a rare condition.
   d. Hoarding symptoms usually occur in the elderly.
   e. Hoarding behaviour is rarely familial.

Answer: a

Hoarding disorder is a new classification in *DSM-5* under obsessive-compulsive and related disorders.

Only 20% of hoarders meet the criteria for OCD.

It is a common condition: studies have shown that the prevalence is between 2% and 6% of the population.

It begins in early in life (between 11 and 15 years), but is more common in older adults.

Almost 50% of people diagnosed with hoarding disorder have a family history of the disorder.

READINGS AND REFERENCES
American Psychiatric Association. *Diagnostic and Statistical Manual of Mental Disorders.* 5th ed. Washington, DC: American Psychiatric Publishing; 2013:247–251.

28. Which of the following statements about disruptive mood dysregulation disorder (DMDD) is true?
   a. The diagnosis of DMDD should be made before age 6.
   b. DMDD is more common in females than in males.
   c. Recurrent temper outbursts occur on average 2 times per week.
   d. Chronic and severe persistent irritability is the core feature of DMDD.
   e. The rates of DMDD among children and adolescents are less than 1%.

Answer: d

DSM-5 describes the features of DMDD as follows:
- Its core feature is chronic, severe, and persistent irritability.
- A diagnosis of DMDD should not be made for the first time before age 6 or after age 18.
- Rates are higher in males and school-age children than in females and adolescents.
- Recurrent temper outbursts occur on average 3 or more times per week. These outbursts are uncommon for age-appropriate development and occur in various settings.
- The 6-month to 1-year period prevalence among children and adolescents probably falls in the 2% to 5% range.

READINGS AND REFERENCES
American Psychiatric Association. *Diagnostic and Statistical Manual of Mental Disorders.* 5th ed. Washington, DC: American Psychiatric Publishing; 2013:156–157.

29. In the context of developmental pharmacokinetics, which of the following is a physiologic characteristic of children, compared to adults, that affects drug action?
   a. smaller body size
   b. less body water
   c. more fat
   d. more plasma albumin to which drugs can bind
   e. bigger volume of distribution

Answer: a

Pharmacokinetics defines drug availability at the site of action. The basic pharmacokinetic processes include absorption, distribution, metabolism, and excretion.

Developmental pharmacokinetics considers age-related physiologic differences that affect the action of drugs.

Compared to adults, children have:
- smaller body size
- greater proportion of kidney and liver parenchyma when adjusted for weight
- more body water
- less fat
- less plasma albumin

These could all result in a lower volume of distribution compared to adults.

READINGS AND REFERENCES
McVoy M, Findling R. *Clinical Manual of Child and Adolescent Psychopharmacology.* 2nd ed. Arlington, VA: American Psychiatric Publishing; 2013.

30. **Which of the following food products should be avoided if a patient is taking irreversible monoamine oxidase inhibitors (irreversible MAOIs)?**
    a. cottage cheese
    b. strawberries
    c. bananas
    d. pineapple
    e. avocados

Answer: e

Irreversible MAOIs include isocarboxazid, phenelzine, tranylcypromine, and selegiline. They interact with foods high in tyramine and certain medications, which can cause hypertensive crisis.

Foods high in tyramine include:
- foods that have been aged, fermented, pickled, cured, or smoked—e.g., many cheeses, beer (especially from tap), wine (especially red), concentrated yeast extract, nonfresh meat (e.g., sausage, salami), yogurt, sauerkraut, fermented soy products (e.g., soy sauce, miso)
- liver (often high in tyramine—best avoided)
- certain fruits and vegetables: broad beans (fava beans), avocado, banana peels, figs, raisins, overripe fruit

READINGS AND REFERENCES
Bhagwagar Z, Heninger GR. Antidepressants. In: Gelder MG, Andreasen MD, López-Ibor Jr. JJ, Geddes R, eds. *New Oxford Textbook of Psychiatry.* Vol 2. 2nd ed. Oxford, UK: Oxford University Press; 2012:1185–1208.

Jacobson MJ, Jacobson SL, Thase ME. Depressive disorders. In: Kupfer DJ, Horner MS, Brent DA, et al, eds. *Oxford American Handbook of Psychiatry.* Oxford: Oxford University Press; 2008:322.

31. Which of the following statements about brain-derived neurotrophic factor (BDNF) is true?
  a. It is involved in short-term memory in adults in all phases of bipolar disorder.
  b. Serum BDNF increases with each episode of depression.
  c. BDNF is related to substance-abuse comorbidity.
  d. Lithium treatment decreases BDNF levels.
  e. Carbamazepine decreases BDNF levels.

Answer: c

BDNF is important to synaptogenesis and neural development, and later neuroplasticity and long-term memory in adults, in all phases of bipolar disorder and its treatment. Serum BDNF decreases with each episode of depression or mania, depending on the severity of the illness. Lithium, valproate, and carbamazepine increase BDNF levels.

Some studies suggest BDNF levels are dependent on genetic factors, environmental factors, and substance abuse.

READINGS AND REFERENCES
Post RM. Lithium and related mood stabilizers. In: Gelder MG, Andreasen MD, López-Ibor JJ Jr, Geddes R, eds. *New Oxford Textbook of Psychiatry*. Vol 2. 2nd ed. Oxford: Oxford University Press; 2012:1199–1207.
Post RM. Role of BDNF in bipolar and unipolar disorder: clinical and theoretical implications. *J Psychiatr Res*. 2007;41(12):979–990. Medline:17239400

32. Which of the following statements about receptor occupancy and its effects on antipsychotic mechanisms is true?
  a. Targeting serotonin 5-HT$_{1A}$ receptors improves cognitive function.
  b. Targeting 5-HT$_{2A}$ receptors improves positive symptoms.
  c. Muscarinic receptors are involved in the sedative effects of antipsychotics.
  d. Orthostatic hypotension is due to the effect of α_2-adrenergic receptors.
  e. The 5-HT$_{2A}$ effects of antipsychotics cause weight gain.

Answer: a

The following are the hypothesized therapeutic and adverse effects of receptor occupancy by antipsychotic drugs:
- dopamine D$_2$ (antagonism or partial agonist effects): reduction of positive symptoms
- serotonin 5-HT$_{1A}$ (full or partial agonist effects): cognitive enhancement, reduction of mood and anxiety symptoms

- serotonin 5-HT$_{2A}$ (antagonism): reduction of negative symptoms, reduction of EPS, reduction of mood and anxiety symptoms
- serotonin 5-HT$_{2C}$ (antagonism): reduction of anxiety symptoms
- adrenergic α$_1$: orthostatic hypotension, dizziness
- adrenergic α$_2$: reflex tachycardia
- histamine H$_1$: sedation, weight gain, and drowsiness
- muscarinic M$_1$ (antagonism): reduction of EPS

READINGS AND REFERENCES
Meltzer HY, Bobo WV. Antipsychotics and anticholinergic drugs. In: Gelder MG, Andreasen MD, López-Ibor JJ Jr, Geddes R, eds. *New Oxford Textbook of Psychiatry.* Vol 2. 2nd ed. Oxford: Oxford University Press; 2012:1208–1227.

33. **Which of the following statements about lamotrigine is true?**
    a. Lamotrigine is thought to act on calcium-channel blockers.
    b. Lamotrigine is metabolized by the liver to an inactive glucuronide conjugate.
    c. The clearance of lamotrigine is not affected in patients with renal impairment.
    d. The majority of rashes induced by lamotrigine are life threatening.
    e. Lamotrigine is structurally related to other antiepileptic agents such as carbamazepine.

Answer: b

Lamotrigine is thought to act by blocking voltage-sensitive sodium channels and by inhibiting the release of glutamate. It is metabolized by the liver and excreted in the urine. It should be used cautiously in patients with renal impairment because its clearance is mainly via the kidneys.

Rash is a common side effect of lamotrigine (10%), which is benign in most cases. Life-threatening rash develops in about 1 in 1000 cases—e.g., Stevens-Johnson syndrome (1% to 2%) and toxic epidermal necrolysis. Other common side effects include: dizziness, headache (> 25%), diplopia, ataxia (22%), blurred vision, nausea, somnolence, and sedation (10%).

Lamotrigine is a phenyltriazine compound, structurally unrelated to other antiepileptic drugs.

READINGS AND REFERENCES
Brennan BP, Harrison G, Pope JR. Antiepileptic drugs. In: Gelder MG, Andreasen MD, López-Ibor JJ Jr, Geddes R, eds. *New Oxford Textbook of Psychiatry.* Vol 2. 2nd ed. Oxford: Oxford University Press; 2012:1231–1240.

Virani AS, Bezchlibnyk-Butler KZ, Jeffries JJ, Procyshyn RM, eds. *Clinical Handbook of Psychotropic Drugs.* 18th ed. Cambridge, MA: Hogrefe Publishing; 2009:197–201.

34. Which of the following medications is most effective in the first-line treatment of antipsychotic-induced akathisia?
   a. propranolol
   b. clonazepam
   c. vitamin E
   d. atropine
   e. amantadine

Answer: a

Propranolol is the first-line medication for treating antipsychotic-induced akathisia.

It is part of a management strategy that includes the following steps:
- Identify the possible causative drug (review medication history).
- Reduce the dose of the drug, or slowly increase it.
- Change to a less EPS-prone drug.
- If symptoms persist, consider propranolol (first) or pindolol, betaxolol, or metoprolol.

READINGS AND REFERENCES
Strassnig M, Rock JE, Patterson KR, Stowell KR. Therapeutic issues. In: Kupfer DJ, Horner MS, Brent DA, et al, eds. *Oxford American Handbook of Psychiatry*. Oxford: Oxford University Press; 2008:1058.

35. Which of the following statements about tardive dyskinesia (TD) is false?
   a. It may be caused by dopaminergic receptor supersensitivity in the basal ganglia.
   b. The most common symptom is perioral movements.
   c. GABA hypofunction leading to enhanced dopamine transmission could be a cause.
   d. The rate of TD is higher in bipolar patients than in schizophrenic patients.
   e. Symptoms of TD cannot be suppressed consciously.

Answer: e

The symptoms of TD can be suppressed consciously.

Symptoms usually start with perioral movements. Other symptoms include axial movements (trunk twisting, torticollis, retrocollis, shoulder shrugging, pelvic thrusting) and limb movements (rapid finger or leg movements, hand clenching).

The pathophysiology of TD is not yet fully understood. Theories include:
- dopaminergic/cholinergic imbalance
- upregulation/supersensitivity of postsynaptic dopamine receptors in the basal ganglia following chronic blockade

- GABA hypofunction leading to enhanced dopamine transmission
- genetic vulnerability

TD tends to develop rapidly, stabilize, and frequently remits, even when medication continues uninterrupted. The symptoms often come and go. Between 5% and 40% of all cases remit (spontaneous remission occurs in up to 90% of mild cases). Some cases, however, require treatment (e.g., switching to clozapine appears to be helpful).

The best prevention strategy is:
- careful use of antipsychotics
- regular monitoring with structured assessment tools such as the Abnormal Involuntary Movement Scale (AIMS)

READINGS AND REFERENCES

Margolese HC, Chouinard G, Kolivakis TT, Beauclair L, Miller R. Tardive dyskinesia in the era of typical and atypical antipsychotics—Part 1: pathophysiology and mechanisms of induction. *Can J Psychiatry*. 2005;50(9):541–547. Medline:16262110

Meltzer HY, Bobo WV. Antipsychotics and anticholinergic drugs. In: Gelder MG, Andreasen MD, López-Ibor JJ Jr, Geddes R, eds. *New Oxford Textbook of Psychiatry*. Vol 2. 2nd ed. Oxford: Oxford University Press; 2012:1208–1227.

Strassnig M, Rock JE, Patterson KR, Stowell KR. Therapeutic issues. In: Kupfer DJ, Horner MS, Brent DA, et al, eds. *Oxford American Handbook of Psychiatry*. Oxford: Oxford University Press; 2008:1062.

36. **Which of the following is seen in moderate to severe intoxication of lithium?**

   a. anorexia
   b. ataxia
   c. abdominal pain
   d. dizziness
   e. slurred speech

Answer: a

Lithium intoxication levels and their symptoms include:
- mild to moderate intoxication:
  - 1.5–2.0 mmol/L
  - symptoms: vomiting; abdominal pain; dry mouth; ataxia; dizziness; slurred speech; nystagmus; lethargy or excitement; muscle weakness
- moderate to severe intoxication:
  - 2.5 mmol/L
  - symptoms: anorexia; persistent nausea and vomiting; blurred vision; muscle fasciculations; clonic limb movements; hyperactive deep tendon reflexes; choreoathetoid movements; convulsions; delirium; syncope; stupor and EEG changes; coma; circulatory failure

Lithium intoxication is a psychiatric emergency requiring medical treatment.

READINGS AND REFERENCES

Fernando SJ, Owen JA, Levenson JL. Psychopharmacology. In: Hales RE, Yudofsky SC, Roberts LW, eds. *The American Psychiatric Publishing Textbook of Psychiatry*. 6th ed. Arlington, VA: American Psychiatric Publishing; 2014:929–1003.

Marangell LB, Martinez JM. *Concise Guide to Psychopharmacology*. 2nd ed. Arlington, VA: American Psychiatric Publishing; 2006:146–147.

Sadock BJ, Sadock VA. *Kaplan and Sadock's Synopsis of Psychiatry: Behavioral Sciences/ Clinical Psychiatry*. 10th ed. Philadelphia: Wolters Kluwer/Lippincott Williams & Wilkins; 2007:1058.

37. Which of the following is not seen in folie à deux?
   a. marked dependence on the primary person
   b. social isolation
   c. low intelligence
   d. psychosis in both principal and associate (always in folie folie simultanée)
   e. association with delusional disorder

Answer: d

Folie à deux (shared delusional order) involves the communication of psychiatric symptoms (usually delusions) from an ill individual to another individual.

The disorder is comorbid with depression, dementia, and mental retardation.

Gralnick describes 4 possible relationships between principal and associate: folie imposée, folie simultanée, folie communiquée, and folie induite.

In folie simultanée, the principal is always psychotic while the associate may or may not be psychotic.

READINGS AND REFERENCES

Gralnick A. *Folie à deux*—the psychosis of association: a review of 103 cases and the entire English literature. *Psychiatric Quart*. 1942;16:230–263.

Munro A. Persistent delusional symptoms and disorders. In: Gelder MG, Andreasen MD, López-Ibor JJ Jr, Geddes R, eds. *New Oxford Textbook of Psychiatry*. Vol 1. 2nd ed. Oxford: Oxford University Press; 2012:624–625.

Oyebode F. *Sims' Symptoms in the Mind: An Introduction to Descriptive Psychopathology*. 4th ed. Edinburgh: Saunders Elsevier; 2008:144.

Volk DW, Morine S, Tew JD, Hosanagar A, Travis MJ, Lewis DA. Schizophrenia and related psychoses. In: Kupfer DJ, Horner MS, Brent DA, et al, eds. *Oxford American Handbook of Psychiatry*. Oxford: Oxford University Press; 2008:268.

38. Which of the following is not part of cognitive behavioural therapy (CBT) for delusions?

a. clarifying delusions as beliefs, not facts
b. empirical testing
c. developing a rationale for questioning delusions
d. challenging the evidence for delusions
e. psychoeducation

Answer: e

The following elements may be used in CBT for delusions:

- clarifying delusions as beliefs, not facts
- developing a rationale for questioning delusions (e.g., relief of distress felt by the patient)
- challenging the evidence for beliefs
- challenging the internal consistency of beliefs
- understanding beliefs as reactions to experience
- assessing delusions and alternative meanings for delusions
- empirical testing

Psychoeducation is a component of CBT in depression.

READINGS AND REFERENCES
Birchwood M, Spencer E. Cognitive behavior therapy for schizophrenia. In: Gelder MG, Andreasen MD, López-Ibor JJ Jr, Geddes R, eds. *New Oxford Textbook of Psychiatry*. Vol 2. 2nd ed. Oxford: Oxford University Press; 2012:1315.

39. Which of the following is a risk factor for suicide in schizophrenic patients?

a. male gender
b. older age
c. feeling anxious
d. social isolation
e. cannabis use

Answer: a

Being male is a risk factor for suicide in schizophrenic patients.

Other factors include: younger age, recent hospital discharge, feelings of hopelessness, and depression. Although substance abuse can increase the risk of suicide in schizophrenic patients, there is no evidence to show that cannabis increases the risk of suicide in schizophrenic patients.

READINGS AND REFERENCES
Sadock BJ, Sadock VA. *Kaplan and Sadock's Synopsis of Psychiatry: Behavioral Sciences/Clinical Psychiatry*. 10th ed. Philadelphia: Wolters Kluwer/Lippincott Williams & Wilkins; 2007:484–485.

40. Which of the following statements about type I alcoholism is true?
a. It is the predominant type of alcoholism in females.
b. The onset is usually before age 25.
c. It has a high genetic component.
d. Parental alcoholism is a risk factor.
e. Parental antisocial behaviour is a risk factor.

Answer: a

Claude Robert Cloninger proposed subgroupings of alcoholism (type I and type II) based on Swedish data.
  Type I alcoholism:
- is more common in females
- has onset later in life
- has more associated psychological factors

  Type II alcoholism:
- is common in males who are younger than 25 and who have high genetic loading
- has significant association with parental alcoholism and parental antisocial behaviour

READINGS AND REFERENCES
Cloninger CR. Neurogenetic adaptive mechanisms in alcoholism. *Science*. April 1987;236:411. Medline:2882604
Cloninger CR, Bohman M, Sigvardsson S. Inheritance of alcohol abuse: cross-fostering analysis of adopted men. *Arch Gen Psychiatry*. 1981:38(8):861–868. Medline:7259422

41. Which of the following statements about body dysmorphic disorder (BDD) is true?
a. Compared to OCD, there is less insight in BDD.
b. The common comorbid diagnosis in BDD is OCD.
c. The mean age at disorder onset is usually after 18.
d. The most common worry of BDD patients is their weight.
e. Suicidal ideation is uncommon in BDD patients.

Answer: a

DSM-5 classifies BDD with obsessive-compulsive and related disorders.

Insight among affected individuals varies widely—from good insight to no insight (delusion)—but is generally poor, and generally worse than in OCD.

Psychiatric comorbidity is common in BDD. The common comorbid condition is major depressive disorder (lifetime prevalence of 75%), followed by social anxiety disorder, OCD, and substance-use disorders.

The point prevalence of BDD is approximately 2.4%. The rates could be higher in certain settings, such as cosmetic outpatient surgeries and dermatology clinics. The mean age at disorder onset is usually 16 to 17. It is important to rule out eating disorders if patients are predominantly focused on weight gain.

Individuals with BDD are more likely to have suicidal ideation and suicidal attempts.

READINGS AND REFERENCES
American Psychiatric Association. *Diagnostic and Statistical Manual of Mental Disorders.* 5th ed. Washington, DC: American Psychiatric Publishing; 2013:242–245.

Dougherty DD, Wilhelm S, Jenike MA. Obsessive compulsive and related disorders. In: Hales RE, Yudofsky SC, Roberts LW, eds. *The American Psychiatric Publishing Textbook of Psychiatry.* 6th ed. Arlington, VA: American Psychiatric Publishing; 2014:431–454.

Phillips KA, Diaz SF. Gender differences in body dysmorphic disorder. *J Nerv Ment Dis.* 1997;185(9);570–577. Medline:9307619

42. Which of the following statements about stalking behaviour is false?

a. Most victims are female.
b. Same-gender stalking is a common problem.
c. Psychotic disorders are relatively frequent in the intimacy-seekers group of stalkers.
d. Research has shown that stalkers are more likely to have OCD.
e. Substance abuse is associated with violence in stalking situations.

Answer: d

Stalking is well studied. Estimates of stalking, which vary according to definition, include:

- victims of stalking: 70% to 80% female
- stalkers: 80% to 85% male
- prevalence: 8% to 22% for women, 2% to 8% for men
- same-gender stalking: common
- substance abuse and stalking: associated with violence
- OCD and stalking: stalking behaviour has an obsessive quality, but the state of mind rarely conforms to a diagnosis of OCD

READINGS AND REFERENCES

Eastman N, Adshead G, Fox S, et al. *Forensic Psychiatry*. Oxford Specialist Handbooks in Psychiatry. Oxford: Oxford University Press; 2012:15–52.

Mullen P. Stalking. In: Gelder MG, Andreasen MD, López-Ibor JJ Jr, Geddes R, eds. *New Oxford Textbook of Psychiatry*. Vol 2. 2nd ed. Oxford: Oxford University Press; 2012:1970–1976.

43. **Which of the following is a neurobiological factor involved in the etiology of depression?**

    a. increased brain volume
    b. increased metabolism in frontal and temporal areas
    c. lack of paid employment
    d. low socioeconomic status
    e. low concentration of 5-hydroxyindoleacetic acid (5-HIAA) in cerebrospinal fluid

Answer: e

Studies have repeatedly found low concentrations of the major metabolite of 5-HT (5-HIAA) in the cerebrospinal fluid of depressed patients and suicidal patients.

The etiology of depression has yet to be fully understood. However, it likely involves biological, psychological, and social factors.

In addition to changes in 5-HIAA levels, other neurobiological factors involved in depression include:

- reduced brain volume of the left hippocampus (structural brain change)
- decreased metabolism in the frontal, temporal, and parietal areas (functional brain change)
- alterations to 3 major monoamine systems: serotonin, norepinephrine, and dopamine

Lack of paid employment and low socioeconomic status are social risk factors for depression, but not neurobiological factors.

READINGS AND REFERENCES

Jacobson MJ, Jacobson SL, Thase ME. Depressive disorders. In: Kupfer DJ, Horner MS, Brent DA, et al, eds. *Oxford American Handbook of Psychiatry*. Oxford: Oxford University Press; 2008:290.

Joyce PR. Epidemiology of mood disorders. In: Gelder MG, Andreasen MD, López-Ibor JJ Jr, Geddes R, eds. *New Oxford Textbook of Psychiatry*. Vol 2. 2nd ed. Oxford: Oxford University Press; 2012:645–650.

44. Which of the following tests cannot be used to assess the memory of a patient with mild cognitive impairment (MCI)?

a. Wechsler Memory Scale, fourth edition (WMS-IV)
b. Rey Auditory-Verbal Learning Tool (RAVLT)
c. California Verbal Learning Test (CVLT)
d. Hopkins Verbal Learning Test (HVLT-R)
e. Stroop Color-Word Test

Answer: e

The Stroop Color-Word Test assesses frontal lobe function. The other tests listed in this answer are commonly used to assess memory.

READINGS AND REFERENCES
Blazer D, Steffens D. *Textbook of Geriatric Psychiatry*. 4th ed. Arlington, VA: American Psychiatric Publishing; 2009:215.

45. Which of the following statements about clonidine is true?

a. Its presynaptic α_2-adrenergic activity increases the release of norepinephrine.
b. Diarrhea is a side effect.
c. It reduces activity levels in ADHD.
d. Hypertension is a known side effect.
e. It can be stopped immediately because it has no discontinuation symptoms.

Answer: c

Clonidine is used to treat hyperactivity and aggression in children, among other conditions (e.g., Tourette syndrome, withdrawal from opioids, posttraumatic stress disorder).

Clonidine is a presynaptic α_2-adrenergic receptor agonist: it decreases the amount of norepinephrine released from presynaptic nerve terminals.

The most common side effects are dry mouth, dry eyes, fatigue, sedation, dizziness, nausea, and hypotension.

It should not be stopped immediately due its abrupt discontinuation symptoms (e.g., increased anxiety, restlessness, tremor, abdominal pain, palpitations, and headache).

READINGS AND REFERENCES
Sadock BJ, Sadock VA. *Kaplan and Sadock's Synopsis of Psychiatry: Behavioral Sciences/Clinical Psychiatry*. 10th ed. Philadelphia: Wolters Kluwer/Lippincott Williams & Wilkins; 2007:997–999.

46. **Among high-risk psychotic youth, which of the following is a predictive factor for progression into a full-blown psychotic disorder like schizophrenia?**
    a. unusual, suspicious, or paranoid thought content
    b. male
    c. good academic performance
    d. intellectual disability
    e. medical illness

Answer: a

Unusual, suspicious, or paranoid thought content is a factor that predicts progression into illness among high-risk youth.
  Other identified factors include:
- familial risk for schizophrenia
- recent deterioration in functioning
- greater social impairment
- history of substance abuse

READINGS AND REFERENCES
American Academy of Child and Adolescent Psychiatry. Practice parameter for the assessment and treatment of children and adolescents with schizophrenia. *J Am Acad Child Adolesc Psychiatry*. 2001;40(7 suppl):4S–23S. Medline:11434484

47. **Which of following is not an etiologic or risk factor for enuresis?**
    a. positive family history
    b. decreased vasopressin production during sleep
    c. reduced nocturnal bladder capacity
    d. psychosocial stressor
    e. lowered arousal threshold

Answer: d

All of the answers listed in this question are risk factors for enuresis, except psychosocial stressors. Other risk factors for enuresis include CNS maturational delay, and psychiatric and neurodevelopmental conditions such as developmental delay and intellectual disability.
  Note the distinction between primary versus secondary enuresis:
- primary enuresis: child has never had a dry period of 6 months
- secondary enuresis: child has been consistently dry for 6 months, but bed wetting is occurring currently (i.e., 2 times per week for 3 months)

READINGS AND REFERENCES
Mindell J, Owens J. *A Clinical Guide to Pediatric Sleep Diagnosis and Management of Sleep Problems*. Philadelphia: Wolters Kluwer/Lippincott Williams & Wilkins; 2010:94–95.

48. Which of the following statements about Wernicke dysphasia is true?

a. The primary deficit is in the mechanism by which words are chosen.
b. There is no defect in the appreciation of the meaning of words.
c. The ability to speak is not impaired.
d. Hearing is impaired.
e. Paraphasic errors are frequent.

Answer: e

Paraphasic errors are among the features that characterize Wernicke dysphasia (also known as primary sensory dysphasia or receptive dysphasia). In addition to these errors, individuals with Wernicke dysphasia use words incorrectly, and their sentences contain errors of syntax and grammar.

Other findings seen in Wernicke dysphasia include:

- primary deficit: comprehension of speech
- hearing: intact, as with pure word deafness
- ability to speak: impaired, presumably because auditory associations or schemas must first be aroused before the efferent speech mechanism can produce speech in a normal manner
- fluency of speech: speech is fluent with no appreciation of the many errors in word choices, syntax, and grammar

Primary motor dysphasia (Broca dysphasia) involves:

- nonfluent speech (primary deficit)
- intact auditory comprehension
- somewhat impaired repetition

READINGS AND REFERENCES
Lishman WA. *Organic Psychiatry: The Psychological Consequences of Cerebral Disorders*. 3rd ed. Oxford: Blackwell Science; 1988:51.

49. Which of the following is a test of perception?

a. Token Test
b. Boston Naming Test
c. Graded Naming Test
d. Bender-Gestalt Test
e. California Verbal Learning Test

Answer: d

The Bender-Gestalt Test assesses perception. Features of this test include:
- focus: primarily a copying test (independent of memory and learning ability)
- procedure: subjects copy 9 simple designs, 1 at a time
- diagnostic utility: type and frequency of errors diagnose neurosis, psychosis, and brain damage

Other perception tests include:
- Visual Object and Space Perception Battery: involves 9 tests for visual perception
- Behavioural Inattention Test: assesses unilateral visual neglect

The Token Test and the Boston Naming Test assess language.
The California Verbal Learning Test assesses memory.

READINGS AND REFERENCES
Lishman WA. *Organic Psychiatry: The Psychological Consequences of Cerebral Disorders*. 3rd ed. Oxford: Blackwell Science; 1988:112–117.

50. Which of the following is an element of structural family therapy?
a. psychoeducation
b. communication training
c. problem-solving training
d. examining hierarchy of power
e. thought diaries

Answer: d

Examining hierarchy of power within a family is one of several elements of structural family therapy, which links problems in a family with the organizational structure of the family. Other important elements of family structure for clinical work include boundaries, alliances, coalitions, and nonverbal and verbal behavioural consequences.

The other answers listed in this question are part of cognitive behavioural therapy (CBT). Other aspects of CBT include contingency contracting and operant-condition training.

READINGS AND REFERENCES
Kay J, Tasman A. *Essentials of Psychiatry*. Chichester, UK: John Wiley & Sons; 2006:890.

Case scenarios (OSCE questions)

CASE 1

You are a senior psychiatry resident who has been asked to see a patient by an emergency room physician.

The patient is a 45-year-old man whom the police have brought to the emergency room (ER). The patient's wife called the police when he threatened to kill her and her lover. The wife, a housewife with 3 children, categorically denies having an extramarital affair. She told the police that her husband recently bought a gun, and that he said she and her lover were "plotting to kill him."

When you assess the patient in the ER, he tells you that he could hear his wife and her lover planning; he believes that they have a device to track his movements. He is angry, paranoid, and suspicious of everyone. He threatens to kill his wife and her lover, and gives you a clear and elaborate plan on how he wants to kill them. On further inquiry about his problem, he admits that he has been using cannabis and alcohol every night to help him relax. While you are waiting for security staff to arrive, the patient leaves the ER.

A. What are your differential diagnoses?
B. What are your immediate steps in the management of this patient?
C. The police escort the patient back to the ER and you admit him to an inpatient psychiatric intensive care unit (ICU). The patient is agitated, paranoid, and suspicious toward you. What would your initial treatment orders be?
D. While in the ICU, the patient becomes acutely psychotic and violent. Some hospital staff request that the patient be jailed. How do you respond?
E. You have treated the patient and he is ready to be discharged to the community. However, he has been charged with uttering threats and a trial date has been set. How would you evaluate whether the patient is fit to stand trial?

CASE 1 NOTES

A. What are your differential diagnoses?
- schizophrenia, paranoid type
- substance-induced psychotic disorder
- major depressive disorder with psychotic features
- schizoaffective disorder
- delusional disorder
- bipolar disorder, most recently manic with psychotic features
- antisocial personality disorder
- psychosis secondary to another general medical condition

B. What are your immediate steps in the management of this patient?
- Call the police to secure the safety of the patient's wife and her alleged lover.
- Consider involuntary status for the patient as per the mental health legislation in your province, as necessary.

C. The police escort the patient back to the ER and you admit him to an inpatient psychiatric intensive care unit (ICU). The patient is agitated, paranoid, and suspicious toward you. What would your initial treatment orders be?
- a safe and controlled environment for the patient, staff, and others, including:
  - an appropriate level of monitoring for the patient
  - adequate security staff
  - removal of potentially dangerous materials
  - isolation of the patient from other patients as much as possible
  - availability of restraints and a seclusion room
- defusing the situation: speak to the patient in a nonprovocative, nonconfrontational manner in a calm voice
- monitoring of vital signs
- lab investigations: serum glucose; complete blood count (CBC); serum chemistry; calcium level; creatinine phosphate level; alcohol and drug screen; liver and thyroid function
- medications: available for oral and intramuscular administration
- information:
  - a complete evaluation interview with the patient if possible: psychiatric history, current mood symptoms, detailed suicide risk assessment, substance abuse history
  - previous chart
  - collateral information from the patient's family and others

D. **While in the ICU, the patient becomes acutely psychotic and violent. Some hospital staff request that the patient be jailed. How do you respond?**
   - Provide empathic support to the staff while following the safety protocols of the hospital. Reassure the staff and other patients that the environment will remain safe.
   - Request increased security presence and, if necessary, get help from the police.
   - Debrief the staff about the resolution of the current situation: make sure the staff are comfortable.
   - Place the patient on one-to-one observation as an assault precaution.
   - Offer medication to control the patient's acute psychotic behaviour.
   - Once the patient is calm (not acutely violent), continue to investigate the cause and precipitants of the violent behaviour.
   - Discuss with the patient the rules of the unit and the consequences of violent behaviour, including the possibility of criminal charges.

E. **You have treated the patient and he is ready to be discharged to the community. However, he has been charged with uttering threats and a trial date has been set. How would you evaluate whether the patient is fit to stand trial?**

The evaluation of fitness to stand trial is based on the McCarty criteria. The patient is fit to stand trial if he:
- has no self-defeating motivation
- understands:
  - the role of court participants: defence counsel, Crown counsel, psychiatrist, judge, jury, defendant, and witnesses
  - the charges
  - the basics of court procedure
  - possible penalties (e.g., sentences, probation)
  - the consequences of unmanageable behaviour
  - possible legal defences
- has the ability to:
  - challenge witnesses
  - communicate with an attorney
  - identify and relate relevant facts
  - plan a legal strategy
  - testify coherently
  - appraise likely outcomes

READINGS AND REFERENCES

Davison SE. The management of violence in general psychiatry. *Advances in Psychiatric Treatment.* 2005;11(5):362–370.

McCarty A, Curran W. *Competency to Stand Trial and Mental Illness.* Rockville, MD: National Institute of Mental Health; 1973.

Petit JR. Management of the acutely violent patient. *Psychiatr Clin North Am.* 2005;28(3):701–711. Medline:16122575

CASE 2

You are working in a clinic. An 18-year-old woman has been referred to you by her family physician for further assessment.

The patient presents to the clinic with her 6-month-old baby, who is asleep in a car seat. She says, "You have to help me: there is something wrong in my head." Her baby starts to cry and she immediately turns to her, checks her, talks to her gently, and rocks the car seat.

The patient says that, over the past 3 weeks, she has been hearing voices in her head. She knows they are not real, but she thinks sometimes that they are voices of the devil, sent by God to torture her for being a "bad person." She also states that the voices tell her somebody will take her baby away. She is embarrassed by the voices, and says that sometimes they become so loud she thinks they are true.

She has never heard voices before. She denies that people are out to get her. However, sometimes when she is walking in the street, she feels some people look at her differently and are sent by God to spy on her.

She has been feeling sad for the past few months, and, although she can care for her baby, she sometimes feels overwhelmed. She has been more tired lately and has not been eating well.

The patient's mother reportedly consumed alcohol while pregnant with the patient. An aunt told the patient that the patient had to stay in the hospital for a week after her birth due to "breathing problems."

As a teenager, the patient drank alcohol excessively, and says her parents had many problems with her. She ran away from home several times. She missed a lot of school and was not passing her courses. She attended an alcohol rehabilitation program for 28 days a few years ago. After that, she quit drinking, but began again when she met her current boyfriend a year ago. She has "tried speed a few times."

The patient denies experiencing voices when she was drinking as a teenager. In fact, she says, she used a lot more drugs then compared to now.

She states an uncle has been in and out of the hospital for "hearing voices and for being crazy." Her mother was hospitalized in a psychiatric unit after a suicide attempt by overdosing on pills 10 years ago. Her father left the home at that time. Her mother was an alcoholic and died from alcohol complications 2 years ago.

When you start to discuss treatment, the patient immediately says that there is no one to help her care for the baby. She is not employed. Her boyfriend is "a loser," the baby's father is "gone," and her only sibling is "using heavy drugs."

A. What are the clinical issues arising from this case?
B. Give the biopsychosocial formulation of this case.
C. What additional information would you like to obtain?
D. What is your differential diagnosis for this patient?
E. What further measures would you order for this patient?

CASE 2 NOTES

A. What are the clinical issues arising from this case?

The key clinical features include:

- 18-year-old single mother
- depressed mood for a few months
- 3-week episode of auditory hallucinations and paranoia; no previous similar episodes
- current substance use: drinking alcohol over the past year and using illicit drugs such as speed (methamphetamine)
- history of alcohol misuse and behavioural disturbances as a teenager
- minimal social support in the community
- responsible for a baby: currently coping, but feels overwhelmed at times

B. Give the biopsychosocial formulation of this case.

This is a case of an 18-year-old woman who was referred by her family physician for further assessment.

BIOLOGICAL FACTORS
PREDISPOSING FACTORS

- strong family history of mental illness
  - maternal uncle: hospitalized numerous times for being "crazy," which indicates a long-standing history of mental health problems
  - mother: history of depression and suicide attempts; research has shown an association between maternal depression and risk of psychopathology in offspring
  - strong family history of alcohol problems
- complications during birth (possible hypoxia)
- prenatal alcohol exposure: predisposes individuals to behavioural, cognitive, and learning difficulties; this may have contributed to her school difficulties as a teenager
- temperament as a child: affects behaviour and response to life situations

PRECIPITATING FACTORS

- current alcohol use
- possible head injury: alcoholics are at risk of head injury; although the history does not indicate head injury, this possibility cannot be ruled out in this case

PERPETUATING FACTORS

- continued alcohol and drug use
- significant family history of alcohol and drug use (mother using alcohol)

PSYCHOLOGICAL FACTORS
PREDISPOSING FACTORS
As an infant and a child, this patient may have suffered compromised attachment to her mother. To develop secure attachment with their primary caregivers, children need caregivers who respond appropriately and sensitively to their needs. Otherwise, they may suffer insecure attachment (3 possible types: insecure-avoidant, insecure-ambivalent, and insecure-disorganized), which can lead to problems with maintaining a stable sense of self and regulating self-esteem.

Risk factors for insecure attachment in this patient include:
- hospitalization for a week following birth
- mother's alcoholism, which may have made the mother unavailable to her daughter during her daughter's early years, and which may have also exposed her daughter to trauma and/or neglect during childhood

PRECIPITATING FACTORS
- death of her mother 2 years ago, which continues to stress her: the loss of her primary caregiver triggered the difficulties she is experiencing
- being a new mother, which has reminded her of the difficulties she experienced growing up with her own mother

PERPETUATING FACTORS
- ongoing conflict with her wish to assume the responsibilities she has, such as caring for her child, and the reality of her capacity to do so: this creates anxiety and she develops her own defence mechanisms to manage anxiety
- drinking alcohol to deal with her difficulties
- limited insight into treatment
- difficulties with relationships (may be related to her difficulty with her childhood relationships): her history is filled with abandonment, and, consequently, she expects to be abandoned and abused by people with whom she has relationships

SOCIAL FACTORS
PREDISPOSING FACTORS
- limited social support during childhood: her father possibly was not available, thus making her mother the primary caregiver
- possible impoverished environment during childhood
- possible limited or inadequate schooling
- exposure to drinking alcohol as a coping strategy during childhood

PRECIPITATING FACTORS
- current unemployment
- current financial difficulties

PERPETUATING FACTORS
- difficulties in maintaining supportive relationships

PROTECTIVE FACTORS
- physical: she is physically healthy
- psychological: reality testing is intact at times (e.g., stating she sometimes knows the voices are not real)
- social: she agreed to the assessment, which demonstrates engagement with the physician

C. What additional information would you like to obtain?

A complete evaluation interview is needed and should cover the following:

- presence of mood symptoms: depressed mood; loss of interest; sleep difficulties; feelings of excessive guilt or worthlessness; anhedonia; loss of energy; poor concentration; decreased or increased appetite; suicidal and homicidal ideation
- presence of manic symptoms: distractibility, racing thoughts, inflated self-esteem or grandiosity, pressure of speech, impulsivity, reckless behaviour
- clarification of psychotic symptoms: presence of any hallucinations, delusions, thought disorder, paranoia
- safety issues: current suicidal and homicidal thoughts, planning, intent, and means (e.g., access to weapons); past suicidal ideation, planning, and attempts
- ability to care for the child: any thoughts to harm the baby; any command-type hallucinations telling her to harm the baby; feeling overwhelmed and unable to care for the child (ask relatives or other reliable informants for additional information, if possible)
- past psychiatric history: previous episodes; past hospitalizations (voluntary and involuntary admissions); previous suicide attempts; history of counselling and medication trials, and compliance with treatment
- family history of psychiatric illness
- medical history: results of recent physical examination and laboratory tests, if available; drug tests; any existing medical problems
- a detailed history of substance use, abuse, and addiction issues
- childhood history: neglect or abuse; whereabouts of other family members and availability to patient; school history; friends; social connectedness
- social history: relationships (current and past), work history, financial resources, social support in the community
- a detailed mental status examination

D. **What is your differential diagnosis for this patient?**
   - psychotic disorder not otherwise specified (NOS)
     + rule out alcohol-induced psychotic disorder
     + rule out primary psychotic disorder
   - major depressive disorder with psychotic features
   - bipolar disorder, most recent episode depressed with mood-congruent psychotic features
   - alcohol abuse
     + rule out alcohol dependence

E. **What further measures would you order for this patient?**
   - collaborative care with current provider; request records from family doctor, psychiatrists, and counsellors
   - laboratory tests: CBC to check for anemia (iron deficiency seen in postpartum women, macrocytic anemia seen in alcoholics); thyroid function tests to check for hypo- or hyperthyroidism; serum electrolytes; drug screen; liver function tests; lipid profile since alcohol can cause dysregulation of lipid metabolism; brain imaging (CT scan)
   - physical examination to rule out organic causes for her current presentation

READINGS AND REFERENCES
Cabaniss DL, Cherry S, Douglas CJ, Graver RL, Schwartz AR. *Psychodynamic Formulation*. Chichester, UK: Wiley-Blackwell; 2013.

CASE 3

You are talking on the phone to a family physician about a 35-year-old man.

This man lives with his wife and his 13-year-old stepdaughter. He recently saw his family physician after having some "unpleasant intrusive thoughts about touching his stepdaughter's genitals and other young girls during the last 6 months." He is extremely ashamed and distressed about these thoughts, and is requesting help to overcome them. On further inquiry about his symptoms, he also admits that he has been checking the locks on his doors frequently and has recently started to check his car for signs of intrusion. Because of his repeated checking behaviour, he is often late for work, which has caused some annoyance with his work manager.

He is married and heterosexually oriented. He reported no recent changes in his sexual relationship with his wife, which was corroborated by her. He has never acted on the intrusive thoughts, has no previous history of psychiatric or developmental problems, and has exhibited no prior deviant sexual behaviour. When time permits, he coaches his stepdaughter's soccer team. He admits to using cannabis on a regular basis, but otherwise he denies any substance use.

At the time of assessment, the man was well groomed and well dressed. On appearance, there were no signs of tremor or abnormal movement. He was cooperative throughout the interview. He articulated clearly and answered questions spontaneously with a normal rate of speech. His affect was depressed and his range of mood reduced. He appeared anxious, but did not show any evidence of thought disorder. He felt the unwanted intrusive thoughts about touching his stepdaughter's genitals were beyond his control and disturbing. He denied having any other intrusive thoughts, images, impulsive urges, or psychotic experiences, such as hallucinations or delusions. He was alert and attentive. He had good insight into his situation.

The family physician is concerned about the man's current presentation, and wants your expert opinion on the risk of the man acting on his intrusive thoughts.

A. What differential diagnoses are relevant to this case?
B. The patient's family physician wants your guidance in differentiating individuals with OCD symptoms from individuals who risk committing sexual offences. How would you advise the family physician?
C. You have completed an assessment of this patient and your impression is that he is suffering from OCD. How would you manage his current presentation?
D. You have treated this patient for 6 months with SSRIs, high doses of clomipramine, and intensive CBT. He has responded very well. However, his illness has strained his relationship with his wife, who is threatening to leave him. He asks for your help. How would you respond?

CASE 3 NOTES

A. What differential diagnoses are relevant to this case?
- obsessive-compulsive disorder (with repugnant obsessions) (OCD)
- major depressive disorder
- substance-induced mood disorder
- psychosis NOS
- pedophilic disorder
- antisocial personality disorder

B. The patient's family physician wants your guidance in differentiating individuals with OCD symptoms from individuals who risk committing sexual offences. How would you advise the family physician?

It is important to reassure the family physician that, in a clinical situation, it may be difficult to assess the risk posed by someone with OCD symptoms and sexually aggressive thoughts. You should thank the family physician for contacting you for your opinion.

The intrusive sexual thoughts of people with OCD may differ from those of sexual offenders in several ways (see the breakdown that follows).

INDIVIDUALS WITH SEXUAL THOUGHTS ARISING FROM OCD	SEXUAL OFFENDERS
Find the thoughts repugnant (ego-dystonic); do not act on them, fantasize about them, or masturbate over them	More likely to use sadomasochistic or pedophilic pornography regularly for pleasure
Typically avoid being alone with, or near, young people	Typically consciously seek out places where children play and opportunities to be alone with children
Try to avoid, neutralize, or suppress intrusive thoughts	Are more likely to engage with intrusive thoughts
Experience frequent intrusive thoughts, which they constantly monitor and try to suppress—this activity dominates their mental life	Experience intrusive thoughts less frequently, and usually in response to specific triggers (e.g., child care)
Experience extreme anxiety, distress, and guilt about intrusive thoughts	Do not experience distress about intrusive thoughts
Seek help (common)	Generally do not seek help

C. You have completed an assessment of this patient and your impression is that he is suffering from OCD. How would you manage his current presentation?

Evidence supports cognitive behavioural therapy (CBT) and pharmacotherapy—e.g., a selective serotonin reuptake inhibitor (SSRI)—as the best available treatment for OCD.

- CBT: exposure and response prevention (ERP); at least 13 to 20 weekly sessions with daily homework
- SSRI: typically at high doses for at least 8 to 12 weeks
  - Note that clomipramine is also highly effective for OCD, but an SSRI is generally tried first because of the more favourable side-effect profile of SSRIs.

D. You have treated this patient for 6 months with SSRIs, high doses of clomipramine, and intensive CBT. He has responded very well. However, his illness has strained his relationship with his wife, who is threatening to leave him. He asks for your help. How would you respond?

It is important to respond to the patient's current issues with his wife. Encouraging positive family relationships, and helping the patient feel understood, greatly enhance the benefits of treatment.

- With the patient's permission, arrange a family appointment for him, his wife, and any other family members.
- Acknowledge his wife's difficulties.
- Education is the first step.
  - Provide information about the illness; particularly emphasize that OCD is a biochemically driven disorder that goes beyond personality issues.
  - Recommend books (e.g., Robert Collie, *Obsessive-Compulsive Disorder: a Guide for Family, Friends, and Pastors*; Herbert Gravitz, *Obsessive-Compulsive Disorder: New Help for the Family*; Karen Landsman, Kathleen Rupertus, and Cherry Pedrick, *Loving Someone with OCD: Help for You and your Family*; website of the International OCD Foundation).
- Encourage the family to join a national or local support group for obsessive-compulsive disorder.

READINGS AND REFERENCES

Koran LM, Hanna GL, Hollander E, Nestadt G, Simpson HB. *Practice Guideline for the Treatment of Patients with Obsessive-Compulsive Disorder.* Arlington, Va: American Psychiatric Association; 2007.

Pallanti S, Quercioli L. Treatment-refractory obsessive-compulsive disorder: methodological issues, operational definitions and therapeutic lines. *Prog Neuropsychopharmacol Biol Psychiatry.* 2006; 30(3):400–412. Medline:16503369

Veal D, Freeston M, Krebs G, Heyman I, Salkovskis P. Risk assessment and management in obsessive-compulsive disorder. *Advances in Psychiatric Treatment.* 2009;15(5):332–343.

CASE 4

You are talking to a patient's wife at your outpatient clinic during an appointment made at the wife's request. In addition to your patient and her, the couple's daughters have also come to the appointment.

Although you have been this patient's psychiatrist for several years, this is the first time you have met with his family. The patient is agreeable to discussing his health-related issues with his family.

He has had problems with alcohol dependence for several years. He was a successful businessman who was involved in a car accident after drinking with work colleagues. He lost his driver's license and eventually lost his business. His alcohol problems have gradually worsened. Life in the family has become restricted: they rarely go out. His wife has a good job and both his daughters are attending the local university, doing extremely well. However, the family finances are slowly dwindling due to the patient's spending on alcohol. His wife is worried about how they will continue to pay for their children's education.

The patient has been hospitalized several times for treatment of complications due to alcohol. He has had residential treatment for alcohol dependence more than once. He has also had treatment as an outpatient, which kept him sober for several months.

When you interview the patient during the family appointment, he complains that his wife nags him unnecessarily about his drinking. He admits that during the last few months he has increased his intake of alcohol, but denies that this is a problem because he drinks "only on the weekends and never during the week." He grew up in the area where he currently lives and meets several childhood friends almost daily at a local bar, but continues to deny that alcohol is a problem for him. When you ask about his alcohol use, he is vague about the actual amount.

His wife thinks his drinking is getting out of control and says they have been arguing about his alcohol problems on a daily basis. She is upset and crying, and both daughters are angry. According to his wife, one daughter has stopped talking to him and isolates herself.

A. How will you proceed initially with his family?
B. One of the patient's daughters insists that he should be "locked up in the hospital for several days" to treat his alcohol problems. How would you address her concerns?
C. The patient's wife is crying, and she asks for your help to admit the patient to hospital. How would you advise her?
D. After a lengthy conversation and assessment, you decide that the patient does not need admission to hospital and could be managed with his family support. Against your advice, the patient wants to begin with "controlled drinking" and then proceed to "complete abstinence." How would you respond to this request?

E. You have almost completed the interview with the patient and his family. His wife asks to speak to you alone and the patient agrees. She confides to you that on several occasions her husband has become physically violent toward her. She shows you several bruises on her arms. What is your view on this?

CASE 4 NOTES

A. How will you proceed initially with his family?

- Welcome everyone to your office and introduce yourself to the patient's wife and daughters.
- Try to develop an empathetic relationship with the family.
- Be aware that the family of someone with a drinking problem may have suffered for years without recognition.
- Encourage the family to talk. Gather information to identify family stresses that may be contributing to the patient's excessive alcohol consumption.
- Address his daughters' concerns and try to understand their difficulties.

B. One of the patient's daughters insists that he should be "locked up in the hospital for several days" to treat his alcohol problems. How would you address her concerns?

It is important to acknowledge:

- the family's difficulties
- the possibility that they have suffered for years without recognition (often the case with a family member who has alcohol dependence)
- the benefit they can get from your advice and understanding
- worries the patient's children may have that arguments between their parents could become physically aggressive

Establish with the daughter that you need to conduct a detailed clinical assessment of her father, and this will determine whether you will treat him as an inpatient or continue to treat him as an outpatient.

Provide the family with information about local support groups (e.g., Al-Anon, community mental health programs).

C. The patient's wife is crying, and she asks for your help to admit the patient to hospital. How would you advise her?

Again, it is important to identify the family's concerns and difficulties.

Describe what you will assess to determine the best course of treatment for the patient (inpatient or outpatient treatment):

- severity of his current psychiatric presentation
- medical complications
- availability of professional support to deal with alcohol problems (community services and outpatient services)
- risk issues, particularly risk of suicide and harm to others
- evidence of acute alcohol withdrawal and risk of alcohol withdrawal seizures or delirium tremens
- cognitive impairment

D. After a lengthy conversation and assessment, you decide that the patient does not need admission to hospital and could be managed with his family support. Against your advice, the patient wants to begin with "controlled drinking" and then proceed to "complete abstinence." How would you respond to this request?

The following principles should guide how you respond:
- The patient needs to make his own decision.
- The patient needs to understand all other treatment options (e.g., complete abstinence, deterrent medications, support through community agencies), and their risks (relapse) and benefits.
- Controlled drinking is more likely to be a successful strategy for patients with good social support.
- Controlled drinking may require a higher level of self-control and commitment than other strategies: for example, the patient needs to limit the number of days of drinking and the number of drinks on any occasion.
- The patient needs to work on developing assertiveness skills and other skills to cope with triggers for drinking.
- The patient needs to agree to regular outpatient follow-up and regular blood tests to monitor γ-glutamyltransferase (GGT) levels.

E. You have almost completed the interview with the patient and his family. His wife asks to speak to you alone and the patient agrees. She confides to you that on several occasions her husband has become physically violent toward her. She shows you several bruises on her arms. What is your view on this?

Violence within an intimate relationship, such as a marriage, is known as intimate partner violence (the preferred term to "domestic violence" or "wife beating").

Some factors to note about intimate partner violence include:
- Marital dysfunction is a common problem in intimate partner violence.
- It is associated with high rates of major depressive disorder and posttraumatic stress disorder in female victims.
- It is associated with excessive alcohol use.
- Couples therapy, and successful treatment of alcohol misuse and dependence, reduces intimate partner violence.

READINGS AND REFERENCES

Chick J. Treatment of alcohol dependence. In: Gelder MG, Andreasen MD, López-Ibor JJ Jr, Geddes R, eds. *New Oxford Textbook of Psychiatry*. Vol 1. 2nd ed. Oxford: Oxford University Press; 2012:447–459.

Heru AM. Intimate partner violence: treating abuser and abused. *Advances in Psychiatric Treatment*. 2007;13(5):376–383.

CASE 5

You are a community-based psychiatrist reviewing one of your long-term patients, a 65-year-old woman with a diagnosis of bipolar disorder.

In the past, the patient had marked manic episodes and major depressive episodes. In recent years, she has been on a combination of lithium, an atypical antipsychotic (quetiapine), and a small dose of an SSRI (sertraline).

The patient was married for 35 years. Her husband died a few months ago from a sudden heart attack. She still grieves her husband's death and finds it difficult to move on with her life. Her 2 daughters live out of town, and, since her husband's funeral, she hasn't spoken to them.

You discuss the anxiety associated with her husband's death. During this conversation, you notice that the patient is slightly confused, her affect is flat, and she speaks with long latencies. She also reports trouble sleeping, frequently getting up during the night, and feeling excessively tired. Usually she is well dressed, but today she is unkempt and her clothing is dishevelled. She also expresses feelings of hopelessness, and says at times she has wondered why she should continue to live after her husband's death. It is customary in your practice for your nurse practitioner to ask patients to complete a full Patient Health Questionnaire (PHQ-9): this patient's score is 20 with 6 PHQ symptoms.

In addition to her psychiatric medications, the patient is taking several other medications: ibuprofen for arthritis, ramipril for hypertension, and omeprazole for gastritis. Recently, her rheumatologist started her on a small dose of steroids to better control her arthritis.

A. What are the differential diagnoses to consider for this patient?
B. You are not sure whether the patient is suicidal. How would you ask her about suicidal intent and plans?
C. What do you think about her PHQ-9 score?
D. A medical student, who is doing an elective with you, wants to know how to differentiate normal grief from prolonged grief disorder. How would you answer?
E. After treating the patient for 10 days in the acute inpatient unit, she is ready for discharge. She is concerned about the long-term side effects of lithium and would like to consider an alternative treatment. How would you get informed consent to start her on an alternative treatment?

CASE 5 NOTES

A. **What are the differential diagnoses to consider for this patient?**
   - major depressive disorder
   - bipolar affective disorder, currently depressed.
   - prolonged grief disorder
   - lithium toxicity
   - hypothyroidism
   - mood disorder, steroid induced

B. **You are not sure whether the patient is suicidal. How would you ask her about suicidal intent and plans?**

   If someone has expressed suicidal ideation, it is important to ask direct and specific questions about suicidal intent and plans:
   - Have you felt that you or others would be better off if you were dead?
   - Do you feel that life is not worth living?
   - Do you wish that you were dead?
   - Have you had specific thoughts about how you might take your own life?
   - What have you thought about as a way to take your life? What other things have you considered?
   - Have you obtained, or do you have access to, pills, poison, medication, or weapons?
   - Have you thought about any other way to kill yourself that we have not discussed (e.g., hanging, jumping from a height)?
   - If you were alone right now, would you try to kill yourself? What about in the near future?
   - Have you attempted suicide in the past?
   - Is there any family history of suicide or attempts?

C. **What do you think about her PHQ-9 score?**

   The PHQ-9 score is calculated based on the number of depressive episodes, a severity score, and a functional assessment.

   The number of depressive episodes is used to help diagnose depression.

   The severity score and functional assessment are taken initially as a baseline, and then monitored to evaluate treatment.

   This patient's score of 20 with 6 PHQ symptoms is suggestive of severe depression.

D. **A medical student, who is doing an elective with you, wants to know how to differentiate normal grief from prolonged grief disorder. How would you answer?**

Normal, or uncomplicated grief, is characterized by the following:
- a broad variability in emotions across individual cases
- variability in its main affects or cognitions (e.g., sadness, despair, loneliness, disbelief, bewilderment), its intensity, and duration across individual cases
- symptoms ranging from mild to profound, occasionally resulting in dysfunction; intermingled painful and positive feelings (e.g., joy, peace, gratitude)
- early transition from acute grief states to integrated reminiscences (deceased more easily called to mind, reality of death acknowledged, return to enjoyable relationships and activities)
- formation of a new symbolic relationship with deceased (accepted back into individuals' lives as deceased)

Prolonged grief disorder is characterized by:
- prolonged or intense grief that is associated with substantial impairment to work, health, and social functioning
- difficulty accepting death, with intense separation and traumatic distress usually lasting well beyond 6 months
- repetitive loop of intense yearning and longing, which become the major focus of individuals' lives
- perceptions that life is over, and that the intense pain will never end

E. **After treating the patient for 10 days in the acute inpatient unit, she is ready for discharge. She is concerned about the long-term side effects of lithium and would like to consider an alternative treatment. How would you get informed consent to start her on an alternative treatment?**

You have a duty to obtain the patient's informed consent for any new course of treatment before starting the treatment. This involves informing the patient sufficiently about:
- diagnosis and prognosis
- the proposed treatment, and its risks and benefits (in this case, you could consider a different mood stabilizer, such as divalproex sodium)
- other possible treatments, and their risks and benefits (in this case, you could consider an atypical antipsychotic as a mood stabilizer)
- the risks of forgoing treatment

READINGS AND REFERENCES

American Psychiatric Association. *Diagnostic and Statistical Manual of Mental Disorders.* 5th ed. Washington, DC: American Psychiatric Publishing; 2013:789–792.

Chehil S, Kutcher S. *Suicide Risk Management: A Manual for Health Professionals.* 2nd ed. Chichester, UK: Wiley-Blackwell; 2012.

Feldman MD, Christensen JF. *Behavioral Medicine: A Guide for Clinical Practice.* 3rd ed. New York: McGraw Hill–Lange; 2008.

Maercker A, Lalor J. Diagnostic and clinical considerations in prolonged grief disorder. *Dialogues Clin Neurosci.* 2012;14(2):167–176. Medline:22754289

Zisook S, Shear K. Grief and bereavement: what psychiatrists need to know? *World Psychiatry.* 2009;8(2):67–74. Medline:19516922

CASE 6

You are seeing a patient in the ER, along with a first-year family medicine resident who is doing an elective with you.

The patient is a 35-year-old man who has a history of using multiple substances and a long-term history of schizophrenia. His illness began when he started a job at a construction company, at age 20. He began to hear voices that told him continuously he was "useless." Around the same time, he also began to believe that his coworkers had planted a video camera to monitor his work. He became increasingly suspicious and paranoid, and after about a year quit his job. He says he couldn't take "the constant monitoring by video cameras." He eventually moved out of his parents' home, because he felt his parents were also monitoring him by video camera. He is now living on his own in a socially deprived area and has more access to street drugs. He attends his community outpatient psychiatric clinic on an irregular basis, where he gets his antipsychotic injection. He uses cannabis regularly and is known to drink alcohol heavily. His recent urine test for drug screening was positive for benzodiazepines.

When you assess him, he is agitated, suspicious, and makes accusations against his family. He occasionally stares blankly during the interview, seeming to respond to his "voices." His concentration is poor, he is easily distracted, his conversation jumps from one topic to another, and he lacks insight into his condition.

A. What are your differential diagnoses in this case?
B. The family medicine resident asks you about the reasons for increased substance use in schizophrenic patients. How would you respond?
C. How would you differentiate a non-substance-induced psychotic disorder from a substance-induced psychotic disorder?
D. What are the possible consequences for this patient of using multiple substances?
E. While you are talking to the family medicine resident, the ER staff calls you urgently because the patient is increasingly agitated and threatening. He refuses to talk to you and makes verbal threats. How do you respond verbally to violent behaviour in this patient?

CASE 6 NOTES

A. What are your differential diagnoses in this case?
- schizophrenia
- psychosis not otherwise specified (NOS)
- substance-induced psychotic disorder
- major depressive disorder with psychotic symptoms

B. The family medicine resident asks you about the reasons for increased substance use in schizophrenic patients. How would you respond?

Hypotheses about the relationship between substance use and established schizophrenia include:
- Substance use is a method of "self-medication."
- Substances can change adverse states induced by either the schizophrenia or its treatment.
- The factors associated with substance use in the general population also affect people with schizophrenia (e.g., availability, cost, facilitation of social interaction, intoxication, relaxation, and peer-group use and acceptance).
- Patients want to "relax" or "sleep more" or reduce the intensity of psychotic symptoms.

C. How would you differentiate a non-substance-induced psychotic disorder from a substance-induced psychotic disorder?

Non-substance-induced psychotic disorders are characterized by:
- psychosis that precedes the onset of substance use
- persistent psychosis (longer than 1 month) after acute withdrawal or severe intoxication
- psychotic symptoms not consistent with the substance used
- psychotic symptoms during periods (longer than 1 month) of abstinence
- personal or family history of a non-substance-induced psychotic disorder

D. What are the possible consequences for this patient of using multiple substances?

Multiple substance use may lead to increased:
- psychotic symptoms
- relapses
- hospitalization and use of health-care services
- risk of tardive dyskinesia
- risk of suicide
- violent behaviour

- family conflict

It may lead to decreased:

- treatment compliance

E. **While you are talking to the family medicine resident, the ER staff calls you urgently because the patient is increasingly agitated and threatening. He refuses to talk to you and makes verbal threats. How do you respond verbally to violent behaviour in this patient?**

Before you talk to the patient:

- Call security as a precaution: you will need backup if the patient becomes violent.
- Make sure you have enough nursing staff available who can employ restraints if needed.
- Arrange for medications that may be needed (benzodiazepines, antipsychotic medications, etc.).

When you talk to the patient:

- Stay calm and controlled.
- Give clear and simple instructions.
- Establish rapport with the patient.
- Don't challenge the patient.
- Admit that you feel frightened: this reality check often defuses rage in agitated patients.
- Encourage the patient to talk about what is upsetting him.

READINGS AND REFERENCES

Lubman DI, Sundram S. Substance misuse in patients with schizophrenia: a primary care guide. *Med J Aust.* 2003;178(9):71–75. Medline:12720527

CASE 7

You are working in a busy inpatient psychiatric unit. You have been called by a nurse to see a 38-year-old man with a 12-year history of schizoaffective disorder.

The patient has become agitated and combative, and has been given 2 haloperidol 10 mg injections. His regular medications include haloperidol deaconate injections (75 mg every 4 weeks), fluoxetine (60 mg per day), and valproic acid (1500 mg per day). He now presents with a temperature of 39°C, blood pressure of 180/100, pulse rate of 112 per minute, and respiration rate of 20 per minute. On further examination, he is confused, diaphoretic, and tremulous. You have ordered some urgent blood tests.

A. What differential diagnoses will you consider for this patient?
B. What investigations you would order for this patient?
C. How will you assess his competency to participate in his treatment?
D. The patient's blood reports show the following values:
   - white blood cells (WBC): 7.8×10^9/L
   - blood culture: pending
   - K^+: 6.1 mmol/L
   - Na^+: 140 mmol/L
   - CPK: 8406 IU/L
   - urine: positive for myoglobin
   - ECG: peak T wave, short QT interval, prolonged PR interval

   What is your next step in the management of this patient?
E. The medical consultant informs you that this is a case of neuroleptic malignant syndrome (NMS). What are the principles of management for this condition?
F. After 10 days, the patient has improved medically. The medical consultant asks for the patient's transfer to the psychiatric floor. How would you respond to this request?
G. The patient's mother asks about restarting the patient on his antipsychotic medications. How would you address her concerns?

CASE 7 NOTES

A. What differential diagnoses will you consider for this patient?
- neuroleptic malignant syndrome
- serotonin syndrome
- viral encephalitis/meningitis
- malignant hyperthermia
- lethal catatonia
- sepsis

B. What investigations you would order for this patient?
- CBC with differentials
- blood cultures
- liver function tests
- renal function tests
- electrolytes; protein, calcium, and phosphate levels
- serum creatine phosphokinase (CPK) levels
- urine myoglobin
- arterial blood gas (ABG)
- coagulation studies
- serum/urine toxicology
- electrocardiogram (ECG)

C. How will you assess his competency to participate in his treatment?

You should provide adequate information to the patient (diagnosis; treatment options, including risks, benefits, and prognosis).

After providing this information, assess his competency with the following criteria:
- Is he able to communicate his choice?
- Does he understand the information you have provided about his current condition?
- Is he able to appreciate the available options and consequences?
- Is he able to make a rational decision?

D. The patient's blood reports show the following values:
- white blood cells (WBC): 7.8×10^9/L
- blood culture: pending
- K^+: 6.1 mmol/L
- Na^+: 140 mmol/L
- CPK: 8406 IU/L
- urine: positive for myoglobin
- ECG: peak T wave, short QT interval, prolonged PR interval

What is your next step in the management of this patient?

This is a medical emergency: the patient has signs of rhabdomyolysis and hyperkalemia with cardiac conduction problems.

- Seek an immediate medical consultation.
- Recommend the patient's transfer to ICU.
- Collaborate with the medical consultant to achieve optimal care for the patient.

E. The medical consultant informs you that this is a case of neuroleptic malignant syndrome (NMS). What are the principles of management for this condition?

- Stop all agents that may be causing the syndrome: in this case, discontinue all the patient's current medications.
- Administer benzodiazepines for acute behavioural disturbances.
- Start supportive measures: oxygen, intravenous fluids (to correct volume depletion and hypotension).
- Control the fever (cooling blankets, antipyretics).
- Take steps to prevent renal failure if rhabdomyolysis is suspected: vigorous hydration; alkalinization of the urine using sodium bicarbonate.
- Start pharmacotherapy to reduce rigidity (e.g., dantrolene, bromocriptine, amantadine).
- Consider electroconvulsive therapy (ECT) if there is no response to the above treatment.

F. After 10 days, the patient has improved medically. The medical consultant asks for the patient's transfer to the psychiatric floor. How would you respond to this request?

- It is important to support the decision of your medical colleague and transfer the patient to the psychiatric floor.
- Reassess the patient's psychiatric condition with careful monitoring of his mental and physical status.

G. The patient's mother asks about restarting the patient on his antipsychotic medications. How would you address her concerns?

- This patient will need antipsychotic treatment because of his long-term history of schizoaffective disorder.
- Monitor the patient closely for residual symptoms and allow adequate time before rechallenging on medications.
- Consider:
    - low dose, low potency oral atypical antipsychotic medication
- Avoid depot medications and high-potency conventional antipsychotics.

- Avoid lithium.
- Continue his valproic acid.
- For all medications:
  - Begin with small doses.
  - Increase the doses very slowly, with close monitoring of temperature, pulse, and blood pressure.
  - Consider monitoring creatine phosphokinase (but note that this is controversial).
  - Closely monitor physical and biochemical parameters: this is effective in reducing progression to full-blown NMS.

READINGS AND REFERENCES

Applebaum PS, Lidz CW, Meisel A. *Informed Consent: Legal Theory and Clinical Practice.* New York: Oxford University Press; 1987: 84–87.

Strassnig M, Rock JE, Patterson KR, Stowell KR, et al. Neuroleptic malignant syndrome: therapeutic issues. In: Kupfer DJ, Horner MS, Brent DA, et al, eds. *Oxford American Handbook of Psychiatry.* Oxford: Oxford University Press; 2008: 1066–1068.

Taylor D, Paton C, Kapur S. *The Maudsley Prescribing Guidelines in Psychiatry.* 11th ed. Chichester, UK: Wiley-Blackwell:110.

CASE 8

You are seeing 35-year-old successful miner at your outpatient clinic. He was referred for a psychiatric assessment by his company employee-assistance program. According to the referral note, the mine manager has concerns about the man's unexplained absenteeism; in addition, the man's colleagues have found him more argumentative and irritable than usual.

The man tells you that his wife left him several months ago, taking their children aged 6 and 14. He is now living alone. He has been partying more than usual and admits that he may have some problems with his alcohol consumption. He was previously treated by his family physician for an episode of depression and still takes some "sleeping pills" prescribed at a walk-in clinic. He has had 2 admissions to a local addiction-treatment facility: both times he was discharged from the treatment program for noncompliance with his treatment regime. He also admits that there is a strong family history of alcohol problems. He is a smoker and drinks at least 5 or 6 large cups of coffee while at work.

He is slightly dishevelled, and you feel that he may have had something to drink this morning. When you ask about this, he dismisses your question and becomes upset. Further assessment reveals that he is tremulous and shaky at times. When you start discussing future treatment plans, he becomes angry, and complains he has received poor treatment services in the past. He accuses his employer and the nurse with the employment assistance program of "having an agenda."

A. How would you do a complete substance-use history of this patient?
B. The medical student who is with you at the time of your assessment asks about the role of screening tools in the assessment of alcohol-related problems. How would you answer this question?
C. After your assessment, you conclude the patient is going through alcohol withdrawal. How would you decide whether to treat him as an inpatient or as an outpatient?
D. What is the role of medication in relapse prevention?
E. At the end of your assessment, the patient becomes angry and irritable. He again blames his multiple treatment failures on "the poor service I've been given in the past." You are also upset, because the patient does not want to follow your advice. What is the psychodynamic explanation for the patient's outburst?

CASE 8 NOTES

A. How would you do a complete substance-use history of this patient?
The principles of a complete substance use history include:
- Ask about all categories of substances, whether or not the patient is currently using them: alcohol, benzodiazepines, cannabis, caffeine, nicotine and stimulants, phencyclidine (PCP), opiates, and hallucinogens (LSD).
- The screening questions for all the substances should include:
    - age at first use
    - frequency of use and amount used (and type used, if relevant)
    - route of administration (if relevant)
    - consequences experienced from the substance use
    - treatment history
    - periods of abstinence and relapse
- After completing the assessment, identify whether the patient fulfills the criteria for intoxication, abuse, dependence, or withdrawal.
- Identify any medical and social complications associated with the patient's current substance use.

B. The medical student who is with you at the time of your assessment asks about the role of screening tools in the assessment of alcohol-related problems. How would you answer this question?

Standardized screening tools are used for screening, diagnostic assessment, and evaluation of severity.

The following commonly available assessment instruments can be used for alcohol-related problems:
- Alcohol Use Disorder Identification Test (AUDIT)
    - 10-item questionnaire with a 0-to-5 score for each question
    - quick to administer and score (about 4 minutes total)
    - a score of 8 or more: reasonably good sensitivity in detecting an alcohol-use disorder
- CAGE questionnaire
    - easy to use; 1 positively answered question has a 90% rate of detecting an alcohol-related disorder
    - involves 4 questions, based on the mnemonic **CAGE**: Have you ever...
        1. Felt you should **c**ut down on your drinking?
        2. Felt **a**nnoyed by criticism of your drinking?
        3. Felt **g**uilty about your drinking?
        4. Felt like taking an **e**ye-opener (a drink first thing in the morning)?

- Michigan Alcohol Screening Test (MAST)
  - useful in assessing the extent of lifetime alcohol-related consequences
- Other screening tools
  - DAST: Drug Abuse Screening Test
  - TWEAK: screening for high-risk drinking during pregnancy
  - CRAFFT: designed for adolescents; covers both alcohol and drugs

C. **After your assessment, you conclude the patient is going through alcohol withdrawal. How would you decide whether to treat him as an inpatient or as an outpatient?**
Recommend inpatient treatment if the assessment shows:
- significant withdrawal symptoms
- very high drinking levels
- serious associated medical or psychiatric illness
- multiple failures as an outpatient
- history of withdrawal seizures or delirium tremens

Recommend outpatient treatment if the assessment shows:
- mild to moderate withdrawal symptoms
- availability of stable home support for the patient
- intact support system providing close monitoring: daily visits to a treatment program or physician's office, in conjunction with other supports such as Alcoholics Anonymous (AA) or other cessation groups

D. **What is the role of medication in relapse prevention?**
Three medications can be used in relapse prevention:
- disulfiram: can be used as a deterrent to alcohol use/abuse
- naltrexone: can be used as an adjunct in the treatment of alcohol dependence
- acamprosate: used for maintenance of abstinence; reduces cravings

E. **At the end of your assessment, the patient becomes angry and irritable. He again blames his multiple treatment failures on "the poor service I've been given in the past." You are also upset, because the patient does not want to follow your advice. What is the psychodynamic explanation for the patient's outburst?**
Transference and countertransference feelings are commonly encountered when treating patients with alcohol-use disorders.

If you keep this in mind, it will help you maintain perspective on negative-transference dynamics.

By recognizing and properly interpreting transference feelings, you improve patient care.

READINGS AND REFERENCES

Kosten TR, Newton TF, Garza II RDL, Haile CN. Substance related addictive disorders. In: Hales RE, Yudofsky SC, Roberts LW, eds. *The American Psychiatric Publishing Textbook of Psychiatry*. 6th ed. Arlington, VA: American Psychiatric Publishing; 2014:735–755.

Sajatovic M, Ramirez L. *Rating Scales in Mental Health*. 3rd ed. Baltimore: Johns Hopkins University Press; 2012.

CASE 9

You receive a consultation request from a surgical colleague regarding a 19-year-old male patient.

When you assess this patient, he gives you a detailed history about his current difficulties. He informs you that since childhood he has enjoyed cross-dressing and likes to play with female friends.

He tells you that he feels disgusted with his genitalia and felt sexual preference toward a young man in his class.

Lately, he has become depressed and has gradually started to withdraw from his university course work. Because of his fear of discussing this issue with his parents, he approached his family physician to ask for a referral to a surgeon to castrate him. His family physician politely refused, so the patient cut his scrotum with a knife, resulting in deep lacerations. He has made an excellent recovery from his wounds. Before his discharge from hospital, the surgical team wants a psychiatric opinion.

A. What is your differential diagnosis for this patient?
B. After an evaluation, you have concluded that the patient has gender identity disorder. What common comorbidities should be considered in this patient?
C. Describe how you would assess this patient.
D. With the patient's permission, you meet with the family. The family is supportive of his condition and they are asking your advice on further management. Describe how you would advise the family.
E. After your consultation with the family and the patient, you receive a phone call from the patient's family physician who feels guilty about his initial refusal to refer the patient to a surgical colleague. He asks your advice on getting further information on gender dysphoric patients. What would you recommend?

CASE 9 NOTES

A. **What is your differential diagnosis for this patient?**
- major depressive disorder
- psychosis/schizophrenia
- gender identity disorder
- personality disorder, especially borderline personality disorder (having transient wishes to change gender as part of an overall identity diffusion during times of stress)
- obsessive-compulsive disorder
- paraphilias

B. **After an evaluation, you have concluded that the patient has gender identity disorder. What common comorbidities should be considered in this patient?**

Consider:
- substance related disorders
- depressive disorders (constant desire to act in their desired gender role may lead to a depressive disorder)
- anxiety disorders
- Cluster B personality disorders
- personality disorder NOS

C. **Describe how you would assess this patient.**

Assessment should be done by a specialist in gender identity disorder or by someone with experience in the management of gender dysphoria.

The patient should have a complete psychosexual evaluation that covers:
- personal and family psychiatric history
- current social circumstances
- his view of his body image
- his expectations, desires, needs
- a detailed medical history
- his family's perspectives (with his permission)

Once the diagnosis is confirmed, assess the patient's:
- depressive symptoms and other comorbid psychiatric conditions, particularly any evidence of delusions which could be centred around his sexual identity
- risk of self-harm and suicidal ideation
- gender development, experiences, feelings; sexual development and maturation; sexuality; relationships
- mental state: do a detailed mental state exam

D. **With the patient's permission, you meet with the family. The family is supportive of his condition and they are asking your advice on further management. Describe how you would advise the family.**

As a psychiatrist, you should be able to provide information to the patient and his family about the management of the patient's gender dysphoric issues, including information about:

- supportive psychotherapy, which can be helpful in both transition goals and providing support with his current situation
- real-life testing: a trial of cross-gender living for at least 3 months
- sex reassignment surgery: this patient has already tried to mutilate his genitals; it may be extremely difficult to engage with any treatment other than sex-reassignment surgery
- long-term psychotherapy: sex-reassignment surgery is irreversible, so these patients need to engage in long-term psychotherapy
- referral to endocrinologists and surgeons to assist him in planning and carrying out his specific goals
- experience with sex reassignment: it is the most widely used and studied treatment for adults with gender identity disorder
- hormonal treatment: a close liaison with an endocrinologist to monitor associated side effects is essential

E. **After your consultation with the family and the patient, you receive a phone call from the patient's family physician who feels guilty about his initial refusal to refer the patient to a surgical colleague. He asks your advice on getting further information on gender dysphoric patients. What would you recommend?**

You should be helpful in providing information to your colleague as this could be a difficult situation for him.

He can also contact an expert from the nearest centre of excellence that specializes in managing gender identity disorders.

Clinicians who are considering providing services to gender dysphoric patients should familiarize themselves with the following guidelines:

- Meyer M, Bockting WO, Cohen-Kettenis P, et al; Harry Benjamin International Gender Dysphoria Association. Standards of care for gender identity disorders, sixth version. *Journal of Psychology and Human Sexuality.* 2002;13(1):1–30.
- American Psychiatric Association, Commission on Psychotherapy by Psychiatrists (COPP). Position statement on therapies focused on attempts to change sexual orientation (reparative or conversion therapies. *American Journal of Psychiatry.* 2000:157(10):1719–1721.

READINGS AND REFERENCES

American Psychiatric Association. *Diagnostic and Statistical Manual of Mental Disorders.* 5th ed. Washington, DC: American Psychiatric Publishing; 2013:451–459.

Becker JV, Perkins A. Gender dysphoria. In: Hales RE, Yudofsky SC, Roberts LW, eds. *The American Psychiatric Publishing Textbook of Psychiatry.* 6th ed. Arlington, VA: American Psychiatric Publishing; 2014:621–702.

Friedman C. Reproductive psychiatry and sexuality. In: Kupfer DJ, Horner MS, Brent DA, et al, eds. *Oxford American Handbook of Psychiatry.* Oxford: Oxford University Press; 2008:528–529.

CASE 10

You are the on-call psychiatrist providing urgent psychiatric care to a hospital ER and to surrounding nursing homes. While you are seeing a patient in the ER, you are urgently paged through the switchboard to speak to a nurse from one of the nursing homes. The nurse is initially frustrated with you, because it takes a half-hour to track you down in the ER. She wants you to see a patient urgently because he is showing disruptive behaviours, including hitting and kicking staff while they are helping him with his activities of daily living (ADLs). These behaviours have escalated over the last few days: he has become quite aggressive and is behaving strangely with staff. The nurse's manager has told the nurse to call you and have the patient transferred to the ER as soon as possible, because the nursing home staff can no longer cope.

You are able to calm the nurse down and establish that she wants you to see a patient in the nursing home. The patient is a 72-year-old man with a history of frequent falls and memory problems. He came to the nursing home almost 2 years ago. While you are going through his medical chart, you notice that a few weeks ago the nursing home family physician requested a psychogeriatric consultation. Unfortunately, no one has seen this order and the student nurse who is accompanying you is extremely apologetic about this mistake.

The patient's medical history includes a stroke 1 year ago that left the patient with right-sided weakness; he has been in a wheelchair ever since and requires some assistance with personal care. He also has diabetes, cataracts, and chronic pain from osteoarthritis in his hips. He remains continent of bowel and bladder function.

The patient is sharing a room with 4 other patients. When you see him, he is in a geriatric chair next to the main nursing station so that he can be under close observation. When you speak to him, he is able to talk to you, though at times you feel he is disoriented and confused. He is weary of living in the nursing home and wants to go back to his apartment. He appears to be sad, and becomes irritable and suspicious when you ask him more questions. He has difficulty producing complete sentences and remembering names, and has limited insight with poor judgement. You perform a mini–mental state examination (MMSE) and he scores 23 out of 30. Physical exam reveals the following:

- temperature: 38.9°C (102°F)
- blood pressure: 100/70
- pulse: 108/min
- respiration rate: 18/min

His psychotropic medications include citalopram and temazepam. His other medications include lansoprazole, metoclopramide, acetylsalicylic acid, and metoprolol. He recently completed a course of ciprofloxacin for a urinary tract infection. He is not allergic to any medication.

When you speak to the nursing home manager, she tells you that he has a daughter who visits him on a regular basis. He also has some friends. His granddaughter, who is a nurse in the same facility, sees him on a daily basis.

A. What are your differential diagnoses for this patient?
B. After assessing the patient, you have decided to transfer him to the hospital. What further investigations would you order?
C. After the patient has been treated for his underlying medical problems, he is still confused—mostly at night—and has become more forgetful. What is your further management?
D. You have confirmed a diagnosis of dementia. The patient's daughter asks whether you could recommend any pharmacological management to stop the progression of the patient's dementia. How would you answer her?
E. The patient and his daughter agree to a trial of donepezil. After 6 months of treatment, the patient shows some improvement. He is no longer depressed. He refuses, however, to continue with donezepil. How would you assess the patient's ability to give informed consent regarding his treatment?

CASE 10 NOTES

A. What are your differential diagnoses for this patient?
- delirium due to medical causes
- dementia (Alzheimer disease, vascular dementia, or Lewy body dementia)
- major depressive disorder with psychotic features
- schizophrenia
- general medical disorders (infection, hypoxia, metabolic abnormalities, fluid and electrolyte imbalance)

B. After assessing the patient, you have decided to transfer him to the hospital. What further investigations would you order?

It is important to carry out all the necessary investigations to come to a proper diagnosis.

The following tests should be ordered:
- complete blood count (CBC)
- electrolytes, calcium, magnesium, phosphate
- blood urea nitrogen/creatinine (BUN/creatinine);
- blood glucose
- liver function tests
- thyroid-stimulating hormone (TSH)
- erythrocyte sedimentation rate (ESR)
- folate and vitamin B_{12}
- blood culture
- urinalysis
- ECG
- chest X-ray
- computerized tomography (CT) scan

C. After the patient has been treated for his underlying medical problems, he is still confused—mostly at night—and has become more forgetful. What is your further management?

His current presentation may indicate cognitive impairment, which needs assessment as follows:

Obtain:
- collateral history: with the patient's permission, talk to his daughter, granddaughter, and family physician about his condition and particularly about his memory difficulties (nature, onset, and progression)
- a detailed psychiatric history

Assess:
- language difficulties (e.g., wording finding, comprehension, reading)
- numerical skills (e.g., money management)
- visuospatial function (dressing, spatial orientation, and constructional abilities)
- cognitive function
- possible behavioural issues associated with dementia
- risks to himself (e.g., wandering) and to others
- possible comorbid psychopathology (depression, psychotic symptoms, anxiety disorders, personality changes)
- patient and family needs, in collaboration with a social worker and an occupational therapist

Perform:
- a physical examination: examine for evidence supporting vascular etiology
- further (repeat) blood tests and other investigations if necessary

D. **You have confirmed a diagnosis of dementia. The patient's daughter asks whether you could recommend any pharmacological management to stop the progression of the patient's dementia. How would you answer her?**

At present, there is no way to cure or stop the progression of dementia. However, some medications (e.g., cognitive enhancers) can slow the rate of decline.

- The currently available cognitive enhancers have been found to modestly improve cognition and function.
- However, when these medications are discontinued, there may be a rapid symptomatic deterioration.

You can provide her with printed information on currently available cognitive enhancers, including donepezil, galantamine, rivastigmine, and memantine.

E. **The patient and his daughter agree to a trial of donepezil. After 6 months of treatment, the patient shows some improvement. He is no longer depressed. He refuses, however, to continue with donezepil. How would you assess the patient's ability to give informed consent regarding his treatment?**

For this assessment, you need to confirm that the patient understands:
- the nature of his condition
- the treatment being offered to him now
- risks and potential benefits associated with this treatment
- treatment options, and their risks and benefits
- the consequences of stopping his treatment plan

If he can understand his current situation, he should be able to make his own decision.

READINGS AND REFERENCES

Meagher DJ, Norton JW, Trzepacz PT. Delirium in the elderly. In: Agronin ME, Maletta GJ. *Principles and Practice of Geriatric Psychiatry.* 2nd ed. Philadelphia: Wolters Kluwer/Lippincott Williams & Wilkins; 2011:383–403.

CASE 11

An Asian patient who is 8 weeks postpartum with her second child is referred to you for an urgent psychiatric assessment during an ER visit. According to her husband, for the first few days after the birth, she was tearful but overjoyed about the baby. Over the next 10 days, however, she reported feeling sad, sleeping difficulties, excessive fatigue, lack of energy, and poor concentration. Lately, she has had frequent obsessive thoughts about the safety of her baby. Prior to her ER assessment, she was seen by her family physician, who diagnosed her with postpartum depression and started her on citalopram (20 mg per day).

She responded well for the first 2 weeks, but has now come to the ER. Her husband is very concerned about her current presentation: she has been saying that the baby is "Satan's son" and that she must get rid of her son to save the world. On mental state examination, she alternates between euphoria and irritability. She appears extremely tired, withdrawn, and suspicious. Her thoughts are often disorganized and incoherent. She stares off intermittently and appears to be responding to auditory hallucinations.

Her husband stays with her throughout the interview. He tells you that she had similar problems after her first baby and was in the hospital for 3 months. After her discharge, she continued to see her family physician. He also informs you they are going through a difficult time with immigration issues. There is a strong family history of depression on her mother's side. She has a very supportive family, which includes her parents and 2 brothers. Her husband indicates that he would do anything and everything to help her.

A. What do you think about her current situation?
B. What is the next step in pharmacological management?
C. After pharmacological treatment is started, the patient improves but continues to have some psychotic symptoms. During a family meeting, you recommend continuing her medications. The patient and her husband insist, however, on stopping the medications because the patient wants to breastfeed. How would you advise them?
D. The patient agrees to continue her medications and decides not to breastfeed. After 4 further weeks of treatment, she is not showing any signs of improvement. What is your next step in her management?
E. The patient's husband asks how to avoid relapses of her condition during future pregnancies. How would you address his concern?

CASE 11 NOTES

A. What do you think about her current situation?

She is experiencing acute psychosis.

First, you need to ensure her safety and the safety of her baby:

- Hospitalize the patient immediately: she should remain in hospital until she is stable.
- Ensure she is not left alone with her baby: she could have supervised daytime visits with the baby.

Next, you need to treat her symptoms of psychosis, agitation, and insomnia with medication.

B. What is the next step in pharmacological management?

The following information should guide your decisions:

- Antipsychotics are typically the first-line treatment for psychosis and agitation.
- Atypical antipsychotics have advantages over typical antipsychotics: mood-stabilizing properties, and lower risk of extrapyramidal symptoms and tardive dyskinesia.
- Olanzapine, quetiapine, and risperidone have longer clinical experience, and more safety data in pregnancy and lactation.
    - Regular monitoring is advised: these medications can cause hyperglycemia, hyperlipidemia, weight gain, and extrapyramidal symptoms.
- Adding benzodiazepines (e.g., lorazepam and clonazepam) to antipsychotics has been found effective in treating insomnia and agitation.

C. After pharmacological treatment is started, the patient improves but continues to have some psychotic symptoms. During a family meeting, you recommend continuing her medications. The patient and her husband insist, however, on stopping the medications because the patient wants to breastfeed. How would you advise them?

It is important to provide continuous psychoeducation to the patient and her husband.

They need to know:

- All psychotropic medications are transferred through breast milk to breastfed infants; however, the effects of some of these medications are believed to be clinically insignificant.
- The benefits of breastfeeding need to be weighed against risks to the infant posed by each psychotropic medication.
- The benefits of medication for the mother may supersede concerns about use of the drug in lactation.
- If she becomes severely ill, too disorganized, or presents a risk to her baby in any way, she should not be left alone with the baby at any time.

It is also important to decide whether the patient is well enough to make her own treatment decisions.

D. The patient agrees to continue her medications and decides not to breastfeed. After 4 further weeks of treatment, she is not showing any signs of improvement. What is your next step in her management?

ECT may be useful at this stage. The number of treatments will depend on the severity of the symptoms.

E. The patient's husband asks how to avoid relapses of her condition during future pregnancies. How would you address his concern?

The couple should be provided with appropriate education and guidance about any future pregnancy.

They should be informed that her illness places future pregnancies in a high-risk category and she is also at high risk of developing psychosis following childbirth.

The patient should be provided with preconception counselling, including a careful review of the risks and benefits of pregnancy, and a treatment plan for ongoing monitoring.

If she is going to be on any psychotropic medications during her antenatal period, the risk of teratogenicity associated with the medication should be carefully balanced against the risks to the mother and the fetus of untreated psychotic or mood symptoms.

After childbirth, her postpartum period should be carefully monitored for the first few weeks for indications of psychosis or mood instability.

Insomnia and irritability can be an early symptom of a mood disorder and can trigger postpartum psychosis. The family should be aware of these triggering factors and the patient should minimize sleep deprivation.

There should be a discussion about any psychotropic medication use postpartum, and risks and options for lactation if appropriate.

Regular psychiatric assessment and monitoring for signs of relapse is necessary.

READINGS AND REFERENCES

Marder S. Treatment of postpartum psychosis. UpToDate. www.uptodate.com. Published 21 October 2013. Accessed 15 May 2013.

Perlis RH, Welge JA, Vornik LA, Hirschfeld RM, Keck PE Jr. Atypical antipsychotics in the treatment of mania: a meta-analysis of randomized, placebo-controlled trials. *J Clin Psychiatry*. 2006;67(4):509. Medline:16669715

Yatham LN, Kennedy SH, Parikh SV, et al. Canadian Network for Mood and Anxiety Treatments (CANMAT) and International Society for Bipolar Disorders (ISBD) collaborative update of CANMAT guidelines for the management of patients with bipolar disorder: update 2013. *Bipolar Disord*. 2013;15(1):1–44. Medline:23237061

Yonkers KA, Wisner KL, Stowe Z, et al. Management of bipolar disorder during pregnancy and the postpartum period. *Am J Psychiatry*. 2004;161(4):608. Medline:15056503

CASE 12

A 15-year-old girl was brought to the ER by paramedics after she was found unconscious in her bedroom. Her foster parents found an empty prescription bottle beside her. It was determined that she took an overdose of pills and required medical admission. She was later admitted to a psychiatric unit. When seen by the admitting psychiatrist, the girl said she took the pills because she wanted to commit suicide. She reported sleep problems and weight loss. She has been missing school because she cannot wake up early enough in the morning. She has been isolating herself and refuses to see her friends. When asked about the future, she stated, "What's the point? Everybody ditched me anyway."

The girl was born prematurely. She weighed 2 kg (4 lb 6 oz) at birth and was in ICU for 4 weeks. She suffered from cocaine withdrawal, because her mother had used crack cocaine and other drugs while pregnant. Her mother was the primary caregiver for the first 3 years of the girl's life, but the girl became a ward of child protection services due to neglect by the mother. At that time, the girl weighed 9 kg (20 lb) and was barely able to make sounds. She was placed in a foster home, where she caught up with her developmental milestones, although delayed. She continues to have some speech and reading problems.

Due to her behavioural disturbances, the girl had to change foster homes several times. She hits her head with her fists when she becomes angry. She ran away from the homes, was not attending school, and was smoking marijuana and drinking alcohol with her peers. She said that 6 months ago, she was sexually and physically abused by a 17-year-old foster brother. She has been transferred to another foster home since then. Her current foster mother has been understanding of her situation and supportive of her.

Attempts to place the girl with her relatives or establish contact with her biological mother have not been successful. The girl's behaviour has been very challenging, and she ends up back in foster homes or group homes. Her mother continues to be addicted to illicit drugs despite numerous rehabilitation treatments.

The girl indicated to the admitting psychiatrist that she has had a hard time contacting her new caseworker to arrange family visits. The foster mother stated that the new caseworker has been in place 5 months, replacing a caseworker who had worked with the girl for the past 5 years. The foster mother said the new caseworker had not been in touch for the past 2 weeks, despite the foster mother's numerous messages expressing concern about the girl. The admitting psychiatrist indicated to the girl and the foster mother that the psychiatrist would contact child protection services, which has custody of the girl, to get their consent for treatment, and to obtain collateral information and discuss the girl's present condition with them.

The girl learned just recently that her biological father died from suicide a few months ago while in prison for drug-related charges. She never met him. Her maternal aunt has depression. The girl had numerous ear infections as a young child. Currently, she does not have any active medical problems. She likes to draw and her work recently won in a school art competition.

A. Give the biopsychosocial formulation for this case.
B. How might the girl's experience of physical neglect and sexual abuse affect her adulthood?
C. Name 2 psychodynamic factors that you should be aware of in treating this patient.

CASE 12 NOTES

A. Give the biopsychosocial formulation for this case.

This is a case of a 15-year-old girl who presented to the ER after she overdosed on pills in a suicide attempt.

BIOLOGICAL FACTORS
PREDISPOSING FACTORS

- significant family psychiatric history
  - mother: drug-related problems
  - father: drug-related problems; suicide
  - maternal aunt: depression
- possible attention, emotional, and cognitive difficulties from birth complications
  - mother's drug use during pregnancy: crack cocaine use by women during pregnancy has been linked to behavioural disturbances in children, including increased irritability and crying
  - mother's physical health during pregnancy: it is important to inquire about this because viral infection and maternal malnutrition have been linked to cognitive and emotional difficulties in children
- temperament: likely insecure
- developmental delays: the girl has speech and reading problems; these and other delays need to be fully assessed, because they could affect her academic performance and contribute to her current mental health issues

PRECIPITATING FACTORS

- possible head trauma from hitting herself when she gets angry

PERPETUATING FACTORS

- ongoing drug-related problems

PSYCHOLOGICAL FACTORS
PREDISPOSING FACTORS

A child develops secure attachment to a primary caregiver who responds appropriately and sensitively to the child's needs. A consistent and reliable parent can model healthy ways to resolve interpersonal conflict and help a child develop a secure sense of self.

Factors that have compromised secure attachment for this girl include:

- 4-week ICU hospitalization as a newborn
- evidence of neglect by mother: when the girl came to the attention of child protection services at age 3, she was underweight and delayed
- placement in numerous foster homes: shows the absence of a consistent parent

The girl now has trouble maintaining a stable sense of self, regulating self-esteem, and developing trusting relationships.

Because of inadequate and inconsistent parenting, she is unable to tolerate separations, and is vulnerable to anxiety and mood symptoms when abandonment is possible. She also has problems with self-regulation, which results in unhealthy coping strategies and impulsive behaviour (hitting her head with her fists, running away, and using illicit drugs).

PRECIPITATING FACTORS
- recent sexual abuse by a foster sibling
- recent death of her father, whom she never met: this triggered feelings about the multiple losses she has experienced in her life; in her perception, the important people in her life, such as her mother, father, and other family members, have abandoned and rejected her
- recent departure of her long-term caseworker: this also emphasized the losses in her life, which were exacerbated by her difficulties in contacting her new caseworker

PERPETUATING FACTORS
- her defence mechanisms of acting out and sublimation: she uses drugs and exhibits impulsive behaviour when angry; at other times, she converts these unacceptable impulses into beautiful art work

SOCIAL FACTORS
PREDISPOSING FACTORS
- placement in numerous foster homes
- possible impoverished environment during her first 3 years of life: her mother likely had a poor relationship with her own family, leaving the mother with little or no social support in the community

PRECIPITATING FACTORS
- recent death of her father
- sexual abuse by a foster sibling
- recent replacement of her caseworker

PERPETUATING FACTORS
- continued involvement with peers who use illicit drugs and alcohol

PROTECTIVE FACTORS
- biological: she is in good physical health and has no prior psychiatric disorder
- psychological: intact reality testing; ability to maintain some superficial relationships
- social: interest in arts such as drawing; support of her current foster mother; collaboration of her psychiatrist in advocating for her individual needs with child protection services

B. **How might the girl's experience of physical neglect and sexual abuse affect her adulthood?**

The girl's childhood trauma of physical neglect and sexual abuse can affect the development of all aspects of adult functioning, including:
- impaired coherent and stable sense of self
- development of self-depreciating or masochistic patterns
- persistent problems with regulation of affect and impulse control, leading to the development of depression, posttraumatic stress disorder, anxiety disorders, or substance abuse
- problems with interpersonal relationships

C. **Name 2 psychodynamic factors that you should be aware of in treating this patient.**

This is a complex case, and treating physicians should be aware of the transference and countertransference phenomenon.

READINGS AND REFERENCES

Cabaniss DL, Cherry S, Douglas CJ, Graver RL, Schwartz AR. *Psychodynamic Formulation.* Chichester, UK: Wiley-Blackwell; 2013.

Sadock BJ, Sadock VA. *Kaplan and Sadock's Synopsis of Psychiatry: Behavioral Sciences/Clinical Psychiatry.* 10th ed. Philadelphia: Wolters Kluwer/Lippincott Williams & Wilkins; 2007.

CASE 13

A 48-year-old man presents to the ER, referred by his family physician for an urgent consultation.

His symptoms include: depressed mood, decreased sleep, decreased appetite, weight loss, fatigue, psychomotor retardation, and excessive feelings of guilt. The man denies having any history of mania or hypomania. On further questioning, it becomes clear that he is exhibiting psychotic symptoms. He believes he is suffering from stomach cancer and, therefore, has stopped eating. He has lost more than 11 kg (24 lb) in the last 2 months. He says he does not want to continue suffering from cancer and expresses severe suicidal ideation. His family physician has investigated extensively for his physical problems and has identified no abnormal findings.

The patient does not abuse substances at present; however, in the past he has been treated for alcohol problems. His medical history includes hypertension and hypercholesterolemia for which he takes medication. He has a strong family history of mood disorders on his mother's side.

His past psychiatric history includes several elements. At 18, he was diagnosed with attention-deficit/hyperactivity disorder (ADHD). He can recall having symptoms like distractibility, irritability, and social anxiety. His first hospital admission was at age 26, after the breakup of his marriage. It lasted 6 months and he was treated with antidepressants (he cannot remember the type). His second hospital admission occurred at age 30, after a sudden onset for no apparent reason. He responded well after a few days of combination treatment with SSRIs and CBT.

You admit him to hospital and try him on a different combination of medication along with intense psychological treatment. He is now taking escitalopram (20 mg per day), quetiapine (200 mg per day), and clonazepam (1 mg 3 times per day), in addition to his antihypertensive and statin. The patient is deteriorating and not responding to the treatment plan. He scored 46 on the Beck Depressive Inventory.

The family is concerned and asks what else can be done.

A. What are the some of the clinical warning signs of treatment-resistant depression in this patient?
B. What additional details about his history of attention-deficit/hyperactivity disorder would you pursue?
C. What is your next treatment option for this patient?
D. After augmentation with other agents, the patient still does not respond adequately to his treatment plan. The family has heard about "electric shock therapy" and asks whether it should be considered. How do you respond?

E. In addition to his treatment-resistant depression, are there any other indications for ECT in this patient?
F. The patient and his mother are very anxious about the possible side effects of ECT. How would you address their concerns?
G. A medical student attached to your team is interested in observing the patient's ECT treatment. What is your advice on this?

CASE 13 NOTES

A. What are the some of the clinical warning signs of treatment-resistant depression in this patient?

- multiple prior episodes
- family history of mood disorders
- prior alcohol abuse or dependency
- suicidal thoughts
- prior failure to respond to a single course of antidepressant or psychotherapy

B. What additional details about his history of attention-deficit/hyperactivity disorder would you pursue?

It is possible that he may have exhibited symptoms of bipolar disorder in addition to symptoms of ADHD.

- When he first presented and was diagnosed with ADHD, did he have any other complaints (e.g., insomnia, flight of ideas, or bursts of goal-directed activity or speech)?
- Is there a family history of bipolar disorder, or more than 1 family member with suicidality or substance-abuse problems?

Note that rapid resolution of depressive symptoms after a few days on an antidepressant is indicative of bipolar II disorder.

C. What is your next treatment option for this patient?

His treatment should be augmented with some other agents: e.g., thyroid hormone (T_3 or T_4), lithium, and bupropion or another antidepressant from a different class such as an SNRI.

Additional augmenting agents to consider include a multivitamin, methylfolate (7.5–15 mg per day), omega-3 (500–1000 mg per day), and vitamin D (1000 IU per day).

Consider an exercise and nutrition program to enhance brain neuropeptide and counteract metabolic syndrome.

D. After augmentation with other agents, the patient still does not respond adequately to his treatment plan. The family has heard about "electric shock therapy" and asks whether it should be considered. How do you respond?

If remission has not occurred after the trials of pharmacological agents, it is appropriate to consider more assertive treatment steps.

ECT can be considered in this patient. The family and the patient should be given more information to decide on ECT.

E. In addition to his treatment-resistant depression, are there any other indications for ECT in this patient?

- severe suicidality
- severe psychosis

F. The patient and his mother are very anxious about the possible side effects of ECT. How would you address their concerns?

Before you consider ECT, it is important to alleviate any anxiety associated with the treatment that the patient may have.

You should provide information about ECT, which should cover:

- the nature of the treatment and a description of the process
- the purpose and benefits of treatment
- the likelihood of success, the risks, and the likelihood of adverse effects, including cognitive impairment
- treatment alternatives and confirmation that these will be available if patient decides not to have ECT
- information on patient rights

You could arrange a family meeting with the patient and his mother to explain the known side effects of ECT.

- They should understand that, as with any treatment, ECT can cause several side effects.
- Some side effects are mild and some are more severe.
- Immediately after ECT, many people have a headache, some aching in their muscles; many feel a little dazed and sick.
- There may be some temporary loss of memory or transient memory loss for the time immediately before and after ECT.
- ECT causes contraction of the jaw muscles: there is a small chance of damage to the tongue, teeth, and lips.
- ECT patients are given a general anesthetic, which has risks. These are small (chance of death or serious injury is about 1 in 10,000).
- Though rare, memory problems can be a longer-term side effect, which can affect social and occupational functioning.
- You could also provide them with written information about ECT.

G. A medical student attached to your team is interested in observing the patient's ECT treatment. What is your advice on this?

It is useful for medical students and other students from different disciplines to observe ECT.

The patient's consent is required (patients should feel no obligation to agree) and their decision should be respected at all times.

READINGS AND REFERENCES

Greden JF, Riba MB, McInnis MG, eds. *Treatment Resistant Depression, A Roadmap for Effective Care.* Arlington, VA: American Psychiatric Publishing; 2011.

The Royal College of Psychiatrists. Information about ECT (electroconvulsive therapy). http://www.rcpsych.ac.uk/expertadvice/treatmentswellbeing/ect.aspx. Published April 2014. Accessed July 2014.

Rudolpher, M. Electroconvulsive therapy, transcranial magnetic stimulation, and vagal nerve stimulation. In: Kay J, Tasman A. *Essentials of Psychiatry*. Chichester, UK: John Wiley & Sons; 2006:922–930.

Thase M, Connolly KR. Unipolar depression in adults: treatment of resistant depression. UpToDate. http://www.uptodate.com/contents/unipolar-depression-in-adults-treatment-of-resistant-depression. Updated June 9. 2014. Accessed July 12, 2014.

CASE 14

As the on-call consultation liaison psychiatrist in a hospital, you are asked to see a 17-year-old girl who has recently attempted suicide. You are seeing this patient on the medical floor.

The patient was admitted to the medical floor 2 days ago after taking a handful of her mother's prescription medications, including amitriptyline, fluoxetine, and an antihypertensive. After taking the medications, she drank almost a bottle of vodka. When she arrived at the ER, she was intubated and managed in ICU. Now, she is medically cleared and the internist would like a psychiatric assessment before discharging her.

When you assess the patient, she tells you that she lives with her mother and 2 siblings, ages 4 and 6. Her father has recently left the family, which has made her mother very upset. The parents have been fighting frequently, something they also did before the separation. They are now consulting a lawyer to resolve their separation issues. The patient has stopped calling her friends, and plays on her computer late into the night. Her grades in school are poor. She feels there is no hope of reuniting her parents. She also feels extremely guilty that she is the cause of her parent's separation. As the oldest child in the family, she feels responsible for her siblings and sometimes feels "I can't fix any of these problems."

On further questioning about her current issues, apart from her overdose issue, she reveals that over the last few years she eats unusually large amounts of food, a habit she has struggled to control. She has gained excessive weight and recently joined a gym, which she attends almost daily and on some days more than once. She is extremely concerned about her appearance and thinks she is "fat."

Her mother has a history of depression and alcohol-related problems, and takes antidepressant medication.

A. How would you assess the patient's overdose attempt?
B. What are your differential diagnoses for this patient?
C. What is your evaluation of her eating habits?
D. A medical student who is working with you asks about the role of psychotherapy in the management of bulimia nervosa. How would you answer this question?

CASE 14 NOTES

A. How would you assess this patient's overdose attempt?

The patient took a significant overdose and should be assessed before discharge to obtain a clear understanding of her suicide risk issues and any protective factors. This will allow you to make a decision about her future management.

Before her assessment

- Confirm with the internist that she is medically cleared and ready for discharge.
- Review her chart.
- If available, review her previous medical records; seek and review, in particular, psychiatric records.

During her assessment

- Seek collateral history from her mother by interview and her family physician by phone.
- It is important to decide whether the patient is at high or low risk of suicide at this time.
- Obtain from the patient a detailed history of her current overdose situation and suicide attempt. Seek details about:
  - circumstances leading to the patient's overdose
  - her intention at the time overdose
  - whether the overdose was a planned or impulsive act
  - any steps she took to prevent being found, or to seek help afterwards
  - whether she regrets her action
  - any continuing thoughts of hurting herself, or any active suicidal intention and plan
    - if present: explore the details and assess the motivation for suicide
  - any past suicidal behaviours, suicide attempts (detected or undetected), aborted suicide attempts, or self-harming behaviours
- It is important to look for the presence of any psychiatric disorders (specifically, depression, personality disorders, psychosis, anxiety disorders, and substance abuse).
- Establish the patient's psychiatric history, and conduct a careful psychiatric mental status examination to identify current psychiatric signs and symptoms.
- Identify other current stresses, including:
  - details of relationship issues with her family
  - other problems (e.g., difficulties about school, finances, legal problems, losses, and social isolation)

B. **What are your differential diagnoses for this patient?**
   - major depressive disorder
   - adjustment disorder
   - borderline personality disorder
   - alcohol- and substance-related disorders
   - bulimia nervosa

C. **What is your evaluation of her eating habits?**
   Some of her behaviours are associated with bulimia nervosa, in particular:
   - eating unusually large amounts of food
   - struggling to control her eating habits
   - excessive exercise (goes to gym almost daily, and sometimes more than once a day)
   - extreme concern about her appearance

D. **A medical student who is working with you asks about the role of psychotherapy in the management of bulimia nervosa. How would you answer this question?**
   Psychotherapy is the key treatment for bulimia nervosa, including:
   - CBT: strong evidence of success treating the core symptoms
   - interpersonal therapy (IPT): shown to be quite effective, although the research database is limited
   - guided self-help (e.g., bibliotherapy, online programs): possible useful first step if CBT is unavailable
   - family counselling: important part of management

READINGS AND REFERENCES

Chehill S, Kutcher S. *Suicide Risk Management: A Manual for Health Professionals.* 2nd ed. Chichester, UK: Wiley-Blackwell; 2012.

Marcus MD, Wilson DV. Eating and impulse control disorders. In: Kupfer DJ, Horner MS, Brent DA, et al, eds. *Oxford American Handbook of Psychiatry.* Oxford: Oxford University Press; 2008:458–459.

CASE 15

The ward manager of a 16-bed inpatient unit is concerned about a 16-year-old girl, who was admitted 3 weeks ago to an eating disorders unit. She has a 3-year history of anorexia nervosa.

The girl's admission weight was 27 kg (60 lb) and her body mass index was 12. Initially, she cooperated well with her treatment plan. In the 2 weeks after parenteral treatment, she was motivated in her treatment plan and started to gain weight. Her last measured weight was 36 kg (80 lb) and her family is extremely happy about the rapid progress.

However, the ward manager is concerned that she appears to have lost motivation over the past 2 days. This morning, the girl reported shortness of breath and tiring easily. The staff did an urgent blood glucose level, which showed 2.2 mmol/L. Her hypoglycemia was corrected, but she became weak, and developed swelling in her legs and generalized muscle weakness. This afternoon, while a nurse was checking her blood pressure, she suddenly collapsed. A code blue was called and the patient was immediately transferred to the medical floor. The nurses on your floor are upset about the whole situation.

A. You have arranged a meeting with the staff to debrief the situation. One of the nursing students asks, "What happened to this patient?"
B. The student nurse asks whether regular monitoring through blood tests could have prevented the syndrome. What regular monitoring may have helped?
C. How can refeeding syndrome be avoided?
D. The patient has been treated for her medical problems and now she is back on the psychiatric floor. A resident who is working with you asks about the role of antipsychotic medications, such as olanzapine, in the management of her condition. How would you respond?
E. What is the role of CBT in this patient's management?

CASE 15 NOTES

A. You have arranged a meeting with the staff to debrief the situation. One of the nursing students asks, "What happened to this patient?"

The patient has experienced refeeding syndrome:
- can happen to patients who are receiving artificial feeding (e.g., fed enterally or parenterally)
- involves a shift in fluids and electrolytes leading to hormonal and metabolic changes
- can cause serious clinical complications:
  - significant change in electrolytes: hypophosphatemia, and other changes (e.g., abnormal sodium and fluid balance)
  - changes in glucose, protein, and fat metabolism
  - thiamine deficiency
  - hypokalemia
  - hypomagnesaemia

B. The student nurse asks whether regular monitoring through blood tests could have prevented the syndrome. What regular monitoring may have helped?

The patient should have had a regular ECG and blood tests for phosphate, magnesium, and potassium levels.

C. How can refeeding syndrome be avoided?
- Refeed slowly.
- Adjust refeeding for the age, nutritional status, and developmental stage of the patient.
- Closely monitor electrolytes, cardiac status, and mental status.
- Establish one-to-one nursing observation for the patient, and ensure refeeding is continuously supervised by staff who know the patient and her laboratory results.
- Consult regularly with a dietitian.
- Consult regularly with the eating disorders program.

D. The patient has been treated for her medical problems and now she is back on the psychiatric floor. A resident who is working with you asks about the role of antipsychotic medications, such as olanzapine, in the management of her condition. How would you respond?

Antipsychotic medication such olanzapine is used in the management of anorexia nervosa.
- It helps to induce weight and also reduce anxiety.
- It is usually started in small doses (2.5 mg).

Note that some patients may refuse to accept olanzapine for fear of weight gain.

E. **What is the role of CBT in this patient's management?**

CBT approaches anorexia nervosa as behaviours (food restriction and avoidance) that have become established habits without direct connection to their initial triggers.

CBT for the disorder involves:

- alliance building, where patients develop therapeutic relationships with their therapists
- self-monitoring and regular homework (core techniques)
- evaluation of the patient's motivation and ambivalence around giving up food restriction and avoidance
- establishing the importance of normal eating and weight-range goals
- teaching the skills of challenging dysfunctional thoughts and of thought restructuring (cognitive restructuring)
- providing psychoeducation including:
    - lifestyle advice on avoiding substances
    - getting regular sleep and reasonable aerobic exercise
- providing family education, including a brief psychiatric history and evaluation of family interaction—this will provide some family therapy

READINGS AND REFERENCES

Garner DM, Vitousek KM, Pike KM. Cognitive-behavioral therapy for anorexia nervosa. In: Garner DM, Garfinkel PE, eds. *Handbook for Treatment of Eating Disorders.* New York: Guilford; 1997:94–144.

Powers PS, Santana CA, Bannon YS. Olanzapine in the treatment of anorexia nervosa: an open label trial. *Int J Eat Disord.* 2002;32(2):146–154. Medline:12210656

Solomon SM, Kirby DF. The refeeding syndrome: a review. *JPEN J Parenter Enteral Nutr.* 1990;14(1):90–97. Medline:2109122

CASE 16

A school teacher has requested to meet with you following an incident at her school involving a 7-year-old boy you recently evaluated.

Your evaluation established that the child exhibits bizarre preoccupations, social withdrawal, social isolation, poor academic performance, and some ritualistic behaviour. He has no interest in other children at school and ignores his sibling at home, who is 4 years old. His speech is limited: he uses only a few phrases. According to his mother, his delivery was difficult and he spent time in ICU after his birth. His development was slow and uneventful.

When he is alone, the child is attached to a favourite toy, which is a "miniature horse." He plays with the horse day and night, and never with other toys. He also shows some compulsive adherence to specific routines and rituals. At school, he has difficulty communicating and interacting with other children, and has occasionally displayed aggressive behaviour. Attempts to calm him are usually met with hostility and, sometimes, temper tantrums.

During a recent aggressive outburst, the child hit another child. The teacher has suspended him from school. The child's mother is upset and not sure how to deal with this situation; she has agreed to your meeting with his teacher.

A. How would you describe the main symptoms of autism spectrum disorder (ASD) to the teacher?
B. The teacher asks, "Why does this child only play with his miniature horse, and never with other children?"
C. The teacher asks how you diagnose autism: are there any specific tests?
D. The teacher recently read somewhere that "there are changes in the age criteria for autism in the new manual of mental disorders." How would you answer her question?
E. A medical student attached to your team asks about the differential diagnosis she should consider while seeing a patient with possible ASD. How would you answer her question?

CASE 16 NOTES

A. **How would you describe the main symptoms of autism spectrum disorder (ASD) to the teacher?**

ASD involves a collection of symptoms, including:
- persistent deficits in social communication and social interactions across multiple settings, such as:
    - deficits in social emotional reciprocity (e.g., difficulties reading others' emotions and signalling their own emotions through body movements and facial expressions)
    - deficits in nonverbal communicative behaviours used for social interaction (e.g., difficulties holding eye contact, difficulties using communication behaviours like pointing or showing)
    - deficits in developing, maintaining, and understanding relationships
- restricted or repetitive patterns of behaviour, interests, or activities, such as:
    - restricted and odd behavioural repertoire (e.g., highly ritualized or repetitive ways of handling objects like sucking, shaking, arranging, or carrying around)
    - stereotyped or repetitive speech, movements, or use of objects (e.g., lining up toys or flipping objects)
    - insistence on sameness, inflexible adherence to routines, or ritualized patterns of verbal or nonverbal behaviour (e.g., extreme stress because of minor changes to routines)

B. **The teacher asks, "Why does this child only play with his miniature horse, and never with other children?"**

This behaviour is characteristic of autism: lack of varied, spontaneous, make-believe play and social imitation.

Children with ASD may:
- line up exact numbers of playthings in stereotyped rituals, without apparent awareness of what the toys represent
- may not engage in pretend play, which usually develops by age 2
- if they develop and engage in pretend play, may have "scripted" pretend play that appears to mimic television or books
- may insist on "sameness" (as in this case) or exhibit perseverative behaviour; changes in routine may trigger upset and tantrums

C. **The teacher asks how you diagnose autism: are there any specific tests?**

There are no specific tests to diagnose autism. The diagnosis is clinical and involves a detailed psychiatric assessment, medical examination, neurological examination, and psychological assessment

The diagnosis of ASD:
- should be suspected in children with abnormalities in social interaction, communication, and behaviour
- usually requires a clinician experienced in diagnosing and treating autism
- involves clinical judgement and evaluation based on standard criteria (e.g., the Diagnostic and Statistical Manual of Mental Disorders or the International Classification of Diseases).

D. **The teacher recently read somewhere that "there are changes in the age criteria for autism in the new manual of mental disorders." How would you answer her question?**

This is correct. *DSM-5* specifies the following age-related criteria for autism:
- symptoms begin in early childhood
- symptoms may not fully manifest until social demands exceed capacity (e.g., during middle childhood years, later adolescence, or young adulthood)

E. **A medical student attached to your team asks about the differential diagnosis she should consider while seeing a patient with possible ASD. How would you answer her question?**

Conditions to consider in a differential diagnosis include:
- selective mutism
- other language disorders
- intellectual disability
- stereotypic movement disorders
- ADHD
- schizophrenia

READINGS AND REFERENCES

American Psychiatric Association. *Diagnostic and Statistical Manual of Mental Disorders.* 5th ed. Washington, DC: American Psychiatric Publishing; 2013:50–59.

CASE 17

You are asked give an opinion on a patient diagnosed with adult ADHD by his family physician. The patient has come to your outpatient clinic accompanied by his mother.

The patient is a 22-year-old part-time worker at a local radio station who has presented with a history of "I need something to help me concentrate and keep me out of trouble with my employers." He reports that he has always experienced difficulties with focusing and completing tasks. His mother reports that, in high school, he struggled to complete his homework and had academic difficulties. The patient also recalls that he easily became bored in class, was often fidgety, and could not sit still. Because of his poor academic performance, he dropped out of school.

When you speak to him alone, he admits to using cannabis on a regular basis, which improves his concentration. He has never had a proper assessment. His family doctor has prescribed a short-term small dose of antidepressants. He gives permission for you to contact his family physician and his school for records.

A. What are the basic steps for diagnosing adult ADHD?
B. What rating scales will you use to come to a diagnosis?
C. What are some common comorbid conditions that could be complicating the diagnosis of adult ADHD in this patient?
D. After 6 months of treatment with a stimulant, the patient has not noticed a major improvement. He recently heard about a new treatment called "metacognitive therapy" and would like more information from you.
E. A resident who is working with you asks about the economic impacts of adult ADHD on society. How would address his question?

CASE 17 NOTES

A. What are the basic steps for diagnosing adult ADHD?
- Obtain a developmental history and attempt to corroborate the information with other sources.
- Symptoms should be consistently present before age 12.
- Assess the impact of symptoms on work, school, relationships (including work colleagues), etc.
- Assess attention, concentration, distractibility, and short-term memory.
- Assess the presence of other psychiatric disorders (e.g., depression, anxiety disorders).
- Assess coping skills, including substance use.

B. What rating scales will you use to come to a diagnosis?
The 4 most commonly used self-reporting scales for ADHD are:
- Wender Utah Rating Scale
- Copeland Symptom Checklist for Attention Deficit Disorders—Adult Version
- Conner's Adult ADHD Rating Scales
- Brown Attention-Deficit Disorder Scale for Adults

C. What are some common comorbid conditions that could be complicating the diagnosis of adult ADHD in this patient?
Adults with ADHD are at significantly greater risk of other psychiatric disorders associated with impaired attention and concentration, disinhibition, and difficulty with task completion, including:
- generalized anxiety disorders
- mood disorders
- bipolar disorder
- intermittent explosive disorder
- antisocial and other personality disorders

D. After 6 months of treatment with a stimulant, the patient has not noticed a major improvement. He recently heard about a new treatment called "metacognitive therapy" and would like more information from you.
Metacognitive therapy is a relatively new treatment and not yet widely available.

The theory underlying it was developed in the early 1990s by psychologists Adrian Wells of the University of Manchester and Gerald Matthews of the University of Cincinnati.

It began as a treatment for generalized anxiety disorder. It is now also used for social phobias, obsessive-compulsive disorder, depression, and schizophrenia.

For ADHD, it uses CBT principles to:
- provide contingent self-reward (e.g., for completing aversive tasks)
- break up complex tasks into manageable parts
- maintain motivation by visualizing long-term rewards

It also incorporates traditional cognitive behavioural methods that challenge problematic thoughts.

E. A resident who is working with you asks about the economic impacts of adult ADHD on society. How would address his question?

The economic impacts of adult ADHD are related to:
- prevalence: reported to be 4.4% (highlights the chronic nature of the disorder)
- possible connection of the disorder to a variety of problems—e.g., occupational difficulties, criminal activity, substance abuse, and traffic accidents
- negative effects on family members—e.g., health, work productivity

READINGS AND REFERENCES

American Psychiatric Association. *Diagnostic and Statistical Manual of Mental Disorders.* 5th ed. Washington, DC: American Psychiatric Publishing; 2013:59–65.

Birnbaum HG, Kessler RC, Lowe SW, et al. Costs of attention deficit-hyperactivity disorder (ADHD) in the US: excess costs of persons with ADHD and their family members in 2000. *Curr Med Res Opin.* 2005;21(2):195–206. Medline:15801990

Miller MC. Metacognitive therapy: a possible new approach for ADHD? Havard Health Blog. http://www.health.harvard.edu/blog/metacognitive-therapy-a-possible-new-approach-for-adhd-201210265458. Published October 26, 2012. Accessed July 4, 2014.

Solanto MV, Marks DJ, Wasserstein J, et al. Efficacy of meta-cognitive therapy for adult ADHD. *Am J Psychiatry.* 2010;167(8):958–968. Medline:20231319

CASE 18

As part of your practice's shared-care approach with the local family health team, you are talking to a family physician concerned about a patient you treat in common.

This patient is a 59-year-old man with a long-standing history of psychotic illness. He recently presented to his family doctor's office with palpitations and syncope. His family doctor ordered an urgent ECG along with some blood tests. The patient's ECG showed some abnormalities, including some arrhythmias.

The patient's sister, who accompanied him to his family doctor's office, reported that over the last 2 months the patient has been isolating himself from his family. He has been talking to himself, not sleeping, and not taking care of his hygiene. When he is well, he is a pleasant, outgoing man who helps his sister.

Since his last discharge from your psychiatric clinic almost 5 years ago, the patient has been continued on his medication by his family physician (haloperidol decanoate, 50 mg monthly intramuscular injection; and lithium 900 mg daily).

You now arrange to see the patient in his family physician's clinic urgently.

In preparation for this appointment, you review the notes on the patient. Before his current problems, he was last seen by his family doctor 6 months ago. At that time, he weighed 70 kg (155 lb) and his body mass index was 27. He was smoking 15 to 20 cigarettes daily, drinking at least 12 units of alcohol per week, and wasn't taking regular physical exercise. His last recorded blood-pressure measurement was 150/95. His diet was mostly prepackaged meals and he was eating relatively little freshly prepared food. His last lipid screen recorded a total cholesterol of 6.2 mmol/L, HDL-C of 0.9 mmol/L, LDL-C of 3.0 mmol/L, and triglycerides of 3.5 mmol/L. However, there is no record of him having been offered lifestyle interventions or lipid-lowering therapy. You could not find any records of blood glucose levels.

According to his family physician's note, the patient was recently started on a course of antibiotics (clarithromycin) for an acute episode of pneumonia, in addition to his monthly haloperidol decanoate injection and lithium. The antibiotics were prescribed by a locum family physician who was caring for the patient during the vacation leave of his regular family physician. The patient is now 1 day away from completing his full course of antibiotics.

A. What would you say to the family physician and his team about this patient's current presentation, particularly about his arrhythmia?
B. What other tests would you order at this stage?

C. His sister is concerned about his current weight and lifestyle. How would you advise her about the long-term complications of these 2 issues?
D. After treatment by the health team, the patient is ready for discharge. His depot injection has been stopped and he has started a different oral atypical antipsychotic medication. What advice would you give his family doctor about follow-up care for this patient?

CASE 18 NOTES

A. What would you say to the family physician and his team about this patient's current presentation, particularly about his arrhythmia?

It is most probably psychotropic-related QT prolongation, which might also explain his palpitations and syncope. He is currently on a long-term antipsychotic injection and was recently started on antibiotics. This may have led to an increase of his QT_c interval on ECG. It is also important to rule out any adverse reaction associated with his antibiotic medication.

Some other medical conditions that could cause palpitations and syncope should also be considered, including cardiac problems, anemia, respiratory causes, pulmonary embolism, and alcohol abuse. If in doubt, it is prudent to consult an internist or cardiologist about his abnormal ECG.

B. What other tests would you order at this stage?

Once he has completed his course of antibiotics, you could repeat his ECG.

Because he is showing an abnormal lipid profile on his blood reports, repeat blood tests are indicated, including lipid screening and fasting blood glucose.

C. His sister is concerned about his current weight and lifestyle. How would you advise her about the long-term complications of these 2 issues?

The patient is at increased risk for general medical conditions. His blood tests are abnormal, which indicate he is at risk for:

- type 2 diabetes
- cardiovascular disease: coronary heart disease, stroke, peripheral vascular disease, dyslipidemia (increased total cholesterol, decreased HDL-C, increased LDL-C, and increased triglycerides)
- hypertension
- certain cancers

Increased weight also adds to the risk of other complications associated with obesity.

D. After treatment by the health team, the patient is ready for discharge. His depot injection has been stopped and he has started a different oral atypical antipsychotic medication. What advice would you give his family doctor about follow-up care for this patient?

Follow-up care should include regular monitoring of:

- smoking status
- weight and waist circumference
- blood pressure

It should also include regular lab work, including:

- fasting lipid panel and glucose level
- urea and electrolytes, including creatinine and GFR

- CBC
- ECG
- prolactin levels
- liver function tests

A family history of cardiovascular disease, hyperlipidemia, and glucose intolerance should be obtained and noted in his medical record.

READINGS AND REFERENCES

Taylor D, Paton C, Kapur S. *The Maudsley Prescribing Guidelines in Psychiatry.* 11th ed. Chichester, UK: Wiley-Blackweel; 2012:27–29.

CASE 19

You have been referred to see an 80-year-old man admitted to the medical floor with a history of chest discomfort. All his medical workup was apparently normal and he is being discharged. However, an internist with an interest in psychiatry feels the patient has an anxiety disorder and would like a psychiatric consultation first.

This man states that he was admitted to hospital 6 days ago from a nursing home because of sudden onset of chest pain, palpitations, and shortness of breath. This is his fourth admission to hospital since his wife's death. He reports reduced appetite and loss of interest in activities he once enjoyed. He attributes his current presentation to the death of his wife. They were together "for 50 years" and he says "it has been very difficult." On further inquiry, he describes a range of worries regarding his current health, finances, and his personal safety at the nursing home.

There is no clear history of falls, seizures, or psychosis according to the notes from his family physician, who saw the patient 1 week ago. Apart from arthritis, for which he takes a small dose of ibuprofen, his medical history was noncontributory to his anxiety symptoms. Regarding his psychiatric history, the patient was prescribed a variety of psychotropic medications in the past, including clonazepam for a long period. This was recently increased and the patient reports that he has been taking extra doses to manage his anxiety symptoms.

A. To confirm a diagnosis of anxiety disorder, what further clinical evaluation should you pursue for this patient?
B. What differential diagnoses would you consider for this patient?
C. What rating scales would you use to assess this patient's anxiety symptoms?
D. What laboratory investigations would you consider for this patient?
E. Your ward social worker is wondering whether this patient would benefit from a trial of CBT. What is your view on this? Name some common difficulties of CBT with older adults.

CASE 19 NOTES

A. **To confirm a diagnosis of anxiety disorder, what further clinical evaluation should you pursue for this patient?**

   Further clinical evaluation should investigate:
   - history of the presenting symptoms: chest pain, palpitations, shortness of breath, and worries regarding his current health, finances, and personal safety at the nursing home
   - characteristics of past symptoms
   - medications and substances used:
     - current medications (clonazepam and other benzodiazepines)
     - over-the-counter medications (including any analgesics, cold medications, and herbal or vitamin supplements)
     - other substances
   - more details about current anxiety symptoms
     - family history of anxiety symptoms
     - evidence of worry, apprehension, fearfulness, and distractibility
     - depressive cognitive themes (e.g., thoughts involving loss, guilt, and failure): anxiety is usually associated with a sense of impending tragedy, trauma, strife, etc.
     - physiologic signs of anxiety (e.g., increased pulse rate, rapid breathing, sweating, trembling)
   - personal history of the patient, to obtain an understanding of his strengths, weaknesses, habits, and coping style in a developmental perspective

   Further clinical evaluation should also include:
   - a detailed mental status examination
   - a physical examination, to rule out any medical issues

B. **What differential diagnoses would you consider for this patient?**
   - acute grief reaction
   - major depressive disorder
   - panic disorder
   - specific anxiety disorder
   - alcohol or other substance abuse
   - posttraumatic stress disorder
   - late-life anxiety and depression
   - acute anxiety
   - dementia

- medical conditions, such as infection
- pathological grief reaction

C. **What rating scales would you use to assess this patient's anxiety symptoms?**

A commonly used observer-rated scale is the Hamilton Anxiety Rating Scale (HAM-A). Its key features are:

- It is a 14-item instrument.
- Clinicians rate the severity of symptoms from none (0) to very severe (4).
- A score of 18 or more suggests clinically significant anxiety.

Self-rated scales can also be used, such as:

- State-Trait Anxiety Inventory (STAI)
    - This is a 40-item instrument.
    - It assesses both transient (STAI-State) and enduring (STAI-Trait) symptoms of anxiety.
- Beck Anxiety Inventory (BAI)
    - This is a 21-item instrument.
    - Patients rate the severity of their anxiety symptoms.

D. **What laboratory investigations would you consider for this patient?**

Laboratory investigations should aim to exclude medical conditions that produce symptoms of anxiety (anemia, endocrine disorders, arrhythmia, and substance abuse) and should include:

- CBC
- ECG
- thyroid function tests
- blood glucose
- blood gases
- drug and alcohol screening

E. **Your ward social worker is wondering whether this patient would benefit from a trial of CBT. What is your view on this? Name some common difficulties of CBT with older adults.**

Along with psychopharmacological interventions, psychotherapeutic interventions have been shown to be effective in older adults.

There are some suggestions that CBT should be modified for older adults to accommodate age-associated memory impairment. Older adults may also have multiple medical problems, which can exacerbate symptoms of mental disorders and cognitive deficits, and they may avoid feedback from CBT sessions to reduce their anxiety.

READINGS AND REFERENCES

Lynch TR, Smoskl MJ. Individual and group psychotherapy. In: Blazer DG, Steffens DC, eds. *The American Psychiatric Publishing Textbook of Geriatric Psychiatry*. 4th ed. Arlington, VA: American Psychiatric Publishing; 2009:523. doi: 10.1176/appi.books.9781585623754.398072.

Wyman, MF. Psychotherapy with older adults. In: Agronin ME, Maletta GJ. *Principles and Practice of Geriatric Psychiatry*. 2nd ed. Philadelphia: Wolters Kluwer/Lippincott Williams & Wilkins; 2011:523.

CASE 20

You are the inpatient psychiatrist at a regional hospital. A family physician from a community 150 kilometres away would like to talk to you about a patient she wants admitted.

The patient is a 28-year-old single man who was diagnosed with schizophrenia at age 21. He currently lives in supported accommodation and attends the family physician's clinic on a regular basis. He has been hospitalized 5 times for his condition, each admission lasting more than 8 weeks. He has had adverse reactions to some antipsychotics in the past. He has not followed his treatment program well, especially during the past 2 years. He continues to have auditory hallucinations and paranoid delusions that are persecutory in nature. He is not depressed, and the physician assures you that the patient does not have any medical conditions. The only concern at the moment is that the patient has not been able hold down a job since his diagnosis.

A. The family doctor thinks this patient would be a suitable candidate for clozapine therapy. What information would you seek from the family doctor to assess the suitability of clozapine for this patient?

B. The family doctor would like to give the patient information about clozapine therapy and its monitoring requirements. How would you advise her?

C. After 17 days of treatment in hospital, the patient is slowly being titrated on clozapine. When you are on the floor, the nurse tells you that she is concerned about the patient's heart rate, which was taken before administering his morning dose. His heart rate was 133 beats per minute (baseline 100 beats per minute). His temperature was 38°C. How would you proceed?

D. After successfully starting the patient on clozapine, he is ready for discharge. You inform the patient's family doctor of the discharge plan and explain the need for her to follow up in the community. She expresses concern that she does not have experience with clozapine. How do you respond?

E. After 12 months on clozapine, the patient has no psychotic symptoms. However, his latest white blood cell count (WBC) was 2100. How would you proceed?

F. The patient's sister contacts you. She would like to know why it took so long for her brother to be offered clozapine therapy. How would you respond?

CASE 20 NOTES

A. The family doctor thinks this patient would be a suitable candidate for clozapine therapy. What information would you seek from the family doctor to assess the suitability of clozapine for this patient?

You should seek information about the following:

- verification of the diagnosis (and consider other differential diagnoses, such as schizoaffective disorder, persistent suicidal or self-injurious behaviour, etc.)
- positive and negative symptoms at the time of diagnosis
- functional impairment at the time of diagnosis
- duration of illness
- history with other antipsychotics (confirm that this patient has failed at least 2 trials with other antipsychotics)
- medications given so far, including (for each medication):
  - name of medication
  - dose
  - side effects experienced if any (especially tardive dyskinesia)
  - patient compliance with medication
  - effectiveness
  - length of time on the medication
- other treatments:
  - psychosocial treatment
- support system in place
- substance-use history:
  - if positive, onset of substance use (before or after onset of psychotic symptoms)
- current symptoms:
  - negative, positive, and cognitive symptoms of schizophrenia
  - symptoms of postschizophrenic depression (to rule this out)
- patient's current risk, particularly of suicide
- current physical health of the patient
  - cardiovascular and hematological diagnoses (especially important)
  - history of bone marrow disease, thrombocytopenia, seizure disorder, deep vein thrombosis, glaucoma, diabetes, etc.
- family history of cardiovascular and hematological diseases

B. **The family doctor would like to give the patient information about clozapine therapy and its monitoring requirements. How would you advise her?**
   Before starting clozapine, the following steps are necessary:
   - a physical examination
   - lab investigations: CBC with differentials, fasting blood glucose, creatinine, urea, electrolytes, bilirubin, alkaline phosphatase, and aspartate aminotransferase (AST)
   - ECG
   - electroencephalogram, if there is any history of seizure disorder
   - a discussion with the patient regarding his treatment-adherence issues
   - registration with a monitoring body, such as the Clozaril Support and Assistance Network (CSAN)
   - a discussion with the patient of informed consent and capacity issues relating to clozapine therapy (patients who agree to treatment with clozapine must complete a consent form)
   - a discussion with the patient about the importance of regular blood monitoring

C. **After 17 days of treatment in hospital, the patient is slowly being titrated on clozapine. When you are on the floor, the nurse tells you that she is concerned about the patient's heart rate, which was taken before administering his morning dose. His heart rate was 133 beats per minute (baseline 100 beats per minute). His temperature was 38°C. How would you proceed?**
   - Examine the patient to rule out any other cause of tachycardia.
   - Check for signs and symptoms of myocarditis, such as flulike symptoms, fatigue, dyspnea, and chest pain.
   - If clozapine-related myocarditis is suspected, consider:
     - urgent blood tests for C-reactive protein (CRP) levels
     - CBC with differentials (eosinophilia)
     - ECG (ST depression)
     - troponin measurement
   - Get advice from a cardiologist.
   - Consider reducing the dose of clozapine and going slower with the titration.

D. You have successfully started the patient on clozapine and he is ready for discharge. You inform the patient's family doctor of the discharge plan and explain the need for her to follow up in the community. She expresses concern that she does not have experience with clozapine. How do you respond?
- Offer to be available to discuss any issues with the doctor regarding the patient's management.
- State that you will enroll the patient in a local medication-management clinic for clozapine.
- Tell the doctor about CSAN.

E. The patient has been on clozapine for the last 12 months and currently has no psychotic symptoms. However, his latest white blood cell count (WBC) was 2100. How would you proceed?
- Consider the safety of continuing clozapine.
- Check for any infection or other medical condition that could lower the WBC count.
- Discuss the blood result with the patient, pharmacist, and CSAN.
- Consider the role of lithium in raising the WBC count.

F. The patient's sister contacts you. She would like to know why it took so long for her brother to be offered clozapine therapy. How would you respond?

You should acknowledge her feelings, but let her know that clozapine is only administered to patients with treatment-resistant schizophrenia.

Patients need a history of unsuccessful treatment in at least 2 trials of other antipsychotics before clozapine is an option. This is because clozapine has severe side effects, including rare, but potentially fatal, agranulocytosis.

Because of clozapine's side effects, some physicians continue to use other second-generation antipsychotics as the agent of choice for treatment-resistant schizophrenia.

Unfortunately, there is at present no way to identify patients with treatment-resistant schizophrenia except through a detailed history. Treatment resistance is a poorly defined concept that has evolved since clozapine's introduction.

Currently, a European research study called CRESTAR is trying to identify clinical tools for predicting which patients are likely to require clozapine therapy, and which are at risk of developing serious side effects from clozapine.

READINGS AND REFERENCES

Kings College London. Clozapine and treatment resistance: CRESTAR. http://www.kcl.ac.uk/iop/depts/ps/research/clinicaltrials/ClozapineandTreatmentResistance-CRESTAR.aspx. Published 2014. Accessed July 10, 2014.

Taylor D, Paton C, Kapur S. *The Maudsley Prescribing Guidelines in Psychiatry.* 11th ed. Chichester, UK: Wiley-Blackwell:69–95.

Contributors

Dr. Peter Ajeuzi, MD, MRCPsych (UK), FRCPC
Consultant child and adolescent psychiatrist, Department of Psychiatry, Health Sciences North, Sudbury, Ontario

Dr. Shabbir Amanullah, MD, FRCPC, MRCPsych (UK)
Adjunct professor, University of Western Ontario, London, Ontario
Lecturer, Dalhousie University, Halifax, Nova Scotia
Consultant psychiatrist, Woodstock General Hospital, Woodstock, Ontario

Dr. Katie Anderson, MD
PGY 2 psychiatry resident, Department of Psychiatry, Health Sciences North, Sudbury, Ontario

Dr. S. Bhagavatula, MD, FRCPC
Consultant psychiatrist, Department of Psychiatry, Health Sciences North, Sudbury, Ontario

Dr. Declan Boylan, MD, FRCPC
Consultant psychiatrist, Department of Psychiatry, Health Sciences North, Sudbury, Ontario

Dr. Popuri Krishna, MD, DPM, ABPN, FRCPC
Consultant psychiatrist, Department of Psychiatry, Health Sciences North, Sudbury, Ontario

Dr. Elendu Okoronkwo, MD, DCP (Ire), MRCPsych (UK), FRCPC, PGDip (London, UK)
Consultation liaison psychiatrist, Department of Psychiatry, Health Sciences North, Sudbury, Ontario

Dr. N. Sanjay Rao, MBBS, MD, FRCPsych, MBA
Cognitive behavioural therapist
Head of Psychiatry, Annapolis Valley Health, Nova Scotia
Associate professor of psychiatry, Dalhousie University, Halifax, Nova Scotia

Dr. Angelita Sanchez, MD, FRCPC
Consultant child and adolescent psychiatrist, Department of Psychiatry, Health Sciences North, Sudbury, Ontario

Dr. K. Shivakumar, MD, MRCPsych (UK), FRCPC, MPH
Consultant psychiatrist, Department of Psychiatry, Health Sciences North, Sudbury, Ontario

Dr. Kristina Sutherland, MD, FRCPC
Consultant psychiatrist, Department of Psychiatry, Health Sciences North, Sudbury, Ontario

DISCLOSURE OF COMPETING INTEREST
The contributors to this book have declared all forms of support received within the 12 months before submission of the manuscript for the book.

Index

A
Abnormal Involuntary Movement Scale (AIMS), and tardive dyskinesia (TD), 165
abuse of children
  and body dysmorphic disorder (BDD), 122
  epidemiology, 112–113
acamprosate
  characteristics and effects, 56–57
  relapse of alcoholism, 206
acute dystonic reaction: characteristics, symptoms, risk factors, 33–34
acute psychosis, and safety, 217
ADAS-cog. *see* Alzheimer Disease Assessment Scale, Cognitive
ADHD. *see* attention deficit hyperactivity disorder
adolescents
  mood disorders, 151–152
  psychotropic medications, 30
  stimulants, 74–75
  substance use screening tool, 205
  trauma-focused cognitive behavioural therapy (TF-CBT), 37–38
  treatment-resistant depression (TRD), 30–31
adrenergic α_1 and α_2, effects of receptor occupancy, 163
adults
  attention deficit hyperactivity disorder (ADHD), 239–240
  consequences of neglect and sexual abuse, 223
  developmental pharmacokinetics, 160–161
aggression
  and clonidine, 171
  psychotropic medications, 30

aging
  changes in, 127–128
  hormonal changes, 118
AIMS. *see* Abnormal Involuntary Movement Scale
Ainsworth, Mary, 145
akathisia, antipsychotic-induced: first-line medication, 164
akathisia, features, 34, 115
Alcohol Use Disorder Identification Test (AUDIT), 204
alcohol withdrawal
  and acamprosate, 57
  and alcoholic hallucinosis, 56
  treatment as in- or outpatient, 205
alcoholic hallucinosis
  features and occurrence, 56
  treatments, 56
alcoholism and alcohol dependence
  assessments, 190
  biopsychosocial factors, 181–183
  clinical issues, 181
  and controlled drinking, 191
  evaluation interview, 183
  family of patient (concerns and difficulties), 190–191
  medications, 205
  patient's requests, 191
  positive family history characteristics, 72
  in pregnancy and with baby, 181
  relapse prevention, 205
  screening tools, 204–205
  type I and type II features, 168
  violence, 205
Alzheimer disease
  drugs and side effects, 121
  and insulin, 118
  pathological features, 114
  protective and risks factors, 158

tools and diagnosis, 158
Alzheimer Disease Assessment Scale, Cognitive (ADAS-cog), cognitive dysfunctions and use, 158
amitriptyline, plasma levels of methadone, 103
amnesia due to diencephalic and hippocampal lesions, characteristics, 40–41
amok, as culture-bound disorder, 78
Angelman syndrome, pairing, 67
anorexia nervosa
  antipsychotics, 233
  cognitive behavioural therapy (CBT), 234
  laboratory findings, 128–129
  monitoring, 233
  poor prognosis, 82
  and refeeding syndrome, 233
  suicide risk, 61
antidepressants
  and carbamazepine, 43
  elderly, 37
  and electroconvulsive therapy (ECT), 102
  number needed to treat (NNT) value, 72
  sexual side effects, 80
  side effects, 35–36, 80, 144
antipsychotic-induced akathisia, first-line medication, 164
antipsychotic-induced weight gain, mechanisms, 115
antipsychotics
  and acute dystonic reaction, 33–34
  for anorexia nervosa, 233
  atypical and typical, 217
  and benzodiazepines (BZDs), 217
  and children, 22
  follow-up care, 243–244
  hypothesized effects, 162–163
  monitoring, 126–127
  and receptor occupancy, 162–163
  risks, 30
  schizoaffective disorder, 201–202
  tardive dyskinesia (TD), 165
  for Tourette syndrome, 68
  use and benefits, 217
anxiety disorder
  and cognitive behavioural therapy (CBT), 247
  differential diagnosis, 246–247
  evaluation, 246

laboratory investigations, 247
rating scales, 247
aphonia, as speech disturbance, 78
apolipoprotein E4 allele, in Alzheimer disease, 158
aripiprazole
  disruptive behaviour disorder, 30
  for Tourette syndrome, 68
arrhythmia, and antibiotics, 243
ASD. see autism spectrum disorder
attachment
  compromising factors, 221–222
  factors, 182
attachment theory
  categories in "strange situation," 145–146
  description, 145
attention deficit hyperactivity disorder (ADHD)
  adults, 239–240
  and bipolar disorder, 226
  children, 72–73
  and cognitive behavioural therapy (CBT), 240
  comorbidities, 239
  diagnosis requirements, 152
  diagnosis steps, 239
  economic impacts, 240
  metacognitive therapy, 239–240
  PATS, 72–73
  and psychiatric disorders, 239
  psychostimulants, 23–24
  rating scales, 239
  symptoms, additional, 226
attenuated psychosis syndrome
  criteria and features, 118–119
  symptoms, 36
author-theory pairings, 69
autism spectrum disorder (ASD)
  behaviour, 236
  characteristics, 110
  diagnosis and tests, 236–237
  differential diagnosis, 237
  symptoms, 236

B
BAI. see Beck Anxiety Inventory
basal ganglia
  and obsessive-compulsive disorder (OCD), 76
  and Tourette disorder, 23
BDD. see body dysmorphic disorder

BDI. see Beck Depression Inventory
BDNF. see brain-derived neurotrophic factor
Beck Anxiety Inventory (BAI), 247
Beck Depression Inventory (BDI), 66
Behavioural Dyscontrol Scale, cognitive functions in elderly, 158
Behavioural Inattention Test, 174
Bender-Gestalt Test, features, 174
benzodiazepines (BZDs)
  and alcoholic hallucinosis, 56
  and antipsychotics, 217
  and γ-aminobutyric acid (GABA) receptors, 15–16
  mechanisms of action, 74
Berne, Eric, 69
bilateral thalamic hyperintensity, and Creutzfeldt-Jacob disease, 70
binge-eating disorder, features, 28–29
bipolar disorder
  and attention deficit hyperactivity disorder (ADHD), 226
  brain-derived neurotrophic factor (BDNF), 162
  characteristics, 67
  differential diagnoses, 193
  early onset, 67
  and hypomania, 21–22
  interpersonal psychotherapy (IPT), 155
  and lithium therapy, 101
body dysmorphic disorder (BDD)
  characteristics, 168–169
  conditions and differential diagnosis, 82
  features, 121–122
bone marrow, changes in aging, 127
borderline personality disorder, features, 113
Boston Naming Test, 174
Bowlby, John, 145
BPRS. see Brief Psychiatric Rating Scale
brain-derived neurotrophic factor (BDNF), importance and functions, 162
brain regions, and obsessive-compulsive disorder (OCD), 76–77
breastfeeding, and medications, 217–218
brief focal psychotherapy, characteristics, 83
Brief Psychiatric Rating Scale (BPRS), 62–63
brief psychotic disorders, characteristics, 75–76
Broca dysphasia (primary motor dysphasia), findings, 173

Brown Attention-Deficit Disorder Scale for Adults, for ADHD, 239
bulimia nervosa
  differential diagnoses, 231
  eating habits, 231
  psychotherapy, 231
  self-evaluation, 29
  suicide risk, 61
bulimia nervosa, acute: interpersonal psychotherapy (IPT), 155
buprenorphine
  vs. methadone, 99
  as opiate antagonist, 16
  use and characteristics, 99
bupropion, sexual side effects, 80
buspirone hydrochloride, action and side effects, 14
BZDs. see benzodiazepines

C
CAG (cytosine-adenine-guanine), and Huntington disease, 108–109
CAGE questionnaire, 204
California Verbal Learning Test, 174
cannabis intoxication
  clinical features and symptoms, 34
  physiologic effects, 42
  withdrawal symptoms, 34
carbamazepine
  brain-derived neurotrophic factor (BDNF), 162
  effects, 75
  hematological side effects, 34–35
  plasma levels of methadone, 103
  side effects, 34–35, 85–86
  teratogenicity, 146
  toxicity and metabolism, 42–43
cardiovascular changes, and physiologic changes, 84–85
cardiovascular system, effect of lithium, 116
case control studies, features, 26
catatonia, and electroconvulsive therapy (ECT), 58
Category Fluency Test, and frontal lobe function, 70
caudate glutamate, and obsessive-compulsive disorder (OCD), 38
CBT. see cognitive behavioural therapy
cells, in central nervous system (CNS), 106–107
central nervous system (CNS)
  benzodiazepines (BZDs), 74

cells in, 106–107
and γ-aminobutyric acid (GABA), 15–16
5-HT receptors and electroconvulsive therapy (ECT), 143
CGG (cytosine-guanine-guanine), and fragile X syndrome (FXS), 109
Chess, Stella, 17
chi-square test, in statistical terminology, 19–20
Child Behaviour Checklist (CBCL), 66
children
  abuse, 112–113, 122
  alcoholism in mother, 181–183
  antidepressants, 35–36
  antipsychotics, 22
  attention deficit hyperactivity disorder (ADHD), 72–73
  autism spectrum disorder (ASD), 236–237
  bipolar disorder and hypomania, 21–22
  body dysmorphic disorder (BDD), 122
  clonidine, 171
  conduct disorder, 68
  developmental pharmacokinetics, 160–161
  disruptive behaviour disorder, 30
  methylphenidate, 72–73
  mood disorders, 151–152
  psychotropic medications, 30
  separation/individualism theory, 59
  stimulants, 74–75
  trauma-focused cognitive behavioural therapy (TF-CBT), 37–38
cholinesterase inhibitors, characteristics, 70–71
chromosomal abnormality, in syndromes, 66–67
Clifton Assessment Procedures for the Elderly, 158
clonidine, characteristics, 171
Cloninger, Claude Robert, 168
clozapine
  follow-up, 252
  and heart rate, 251
  and schizophrenia, 250–251, 252
  suitability information, 250
  tests and monitoring, 251
  treatment features, restrictions, and side effects, 116–117, 252
  white blood cell count, 252
CNS. *see* central nervous system
cocaine, effects and dependence, 102–103
cognitive behavioural therapy (CBT)
  and anorexia nervosa, 234
  and anxiety disorder, 247
  and attention deficit hyperactivity disorder (ADHD), 240
  and bulimia nervosa, 231
  and cognitive errors, 41
  and delusions, 167
  and elderly, 247
  elements, 174
  for obsessive-compulsive disorder (OCD), 73–74, 187
cognitive error, identification, 41
Cognitive Estimate Test, and frontal lobe function, 70
cognitive functions
  changes in elderly, 129
  psychometric tests, 157–158
cognitive impairment, assessment, 213–214
cognitive impairment (mild), signs, 81
Cognitive Performance Test, 158
combined pharmacological and psychotherapy treatment, usefulness, 102
competence, of patient, 124–125, 200
complex partial seizure disorder, and carbamazepine, 42–43
compulsion and obsession, causes, 41–42
computed tomography (CT), fluctuating cognitive impairment, 27
conduct disorder
  features, 119
  genetic traits, 22
  kleptomania, 125–126
  parents' conditions, 68
Conner's Adult ADHD Rating Scales, 239
Conners rating scale, 66
controlled drinking, as strategy, 191
conversion disorder, in *DSM-5*, 19
Copeland Symptom Checklist for Attention Deficit Disorders, 239
correlation coefficient, as statistical concept, 149
cortical dementia, features, 65
cortisol, and hormonal changes in aging, 118
CRAFFT (drug-abuse screening test), 205
Creutzfeldt-Jacob disease, and bilateral thalamic hyperintensity, 70
cri du chat syndrome, pairing, 67
cryptographia, as speech disturbance, 78

INDEX

cryptolalia, as speech disturbance, 78
CT. *see* computed tomography
culture-bound disorders, types and descriptions, 77–78
cytosine-adenine-guanine. *see* CAG
cytosine-guanine-guanine. *see* CGG

D

D_2 receptor antagonists, for Tourette syndrome, 68
DAST: Drug Abuse Screening Test, 205
death, stages of reaction, 24
delirium
   hormonal changes in aging, 118
   symptoms, 79–80
delusions
   characteristics, 79
   and cognitive behavioural therapy (CBT), 167
   and schizophrenia, 124
dementia
   characteristics, 126
   donepezil, 214
   progression and medication, 214
   risk factors, 114–115
   symptoms, 79–80
   tools and diagnosis, 158
Dementia Rating Scale, 158
dementia with Lewy bodies (DLB)
   features, 27–28, 64
   findings, 64
depersonalization disorder, characteristics, 156–157
depression. *see also* treatment-resistant depression
   brain-derived neurotrophic factor (BDNF), 162
   characteristics, 126
   chronicity factors, 36–37
   competence of patient, 124–125
   differential diagnoses, 193
   and electroconvulsive therapy (ECT), 58
   and Hamilton Depression Rating Scale (HAM-D), 107
   hormonal changes in aging, 118
   PHQ-9 score, 193
   and postpartum psychiatric disorders, 122
   scale sensitivity and specificity, 123–124
   and selective serotonin reuptake inhibitors (SSRIs), 144
   suicide risk, 60–61

depression, etiology of: neurobiological and other factors, 170
depressive disorder, combined pharmacological and psychotherapy treatment, 102
depressive disorder with atypical features, signs, 127
depressive disorder with melancholic features. *see* melancholic depression
desipramine, plasma levels of methadone, 103
developmental pharmacokinetics, physiologic characteristics, 160–161
diencephalic lesions, and amnesia, 40–41
disruptive behaviour disorder, psychotropic medications, 30
disruptive behaviours, nursing home patient
   detailed management, 213–214
   differential diagnoses, 213
   investigations, 213
disruptive mood dysregulation disorder (DMDD), features, 160
disulfiram, relapse of alcoholism, 206
DLB. *see* dementia with Lewy bodies
DMDD. *see* disruptive mood dysregulation disorder
domestic violence, factors, 191
donepezil
   for Alzheimer disease, 121
   as cholinesterase inhibitor, 71
   for dementia, 214
   use and side effects, 121
dopamine D_2, effects of receptor occupancy, 162
Down syndrome
   and intellectual disability, 151
   pairing, 66
dream work, mechanisms, 155
drug-induced hepatotoxicity, risk factors and causes, 104–105
DSM-5
   alcoholic hallucinosis, 56
   attention deficit hyperactivity disorder (ADHD), 152
   attenuated psychosis syndrome, 36, 118–119
   autism spectrum disorder (ASD), 237
   binge-eating disorder, 28–29
   body dysmorphic disorder (BDD), 168
   brief psychotic disorders, 76

conduct disorder, 119
depersonalization disorder, 156
disruptive mood dysregulation disorder (DMDD), 160
enuresis, 152
hoarding disorder, 159
intellectual disability, 150
melancholic depression, 79
obsessive-compulsive disorder (OCD), 100
obsessive-compulsive personality disorder (OCPD), 100
opioid intoxication, 25
persistent depressive disorder (PDD), 110–111
phencyclidine intoxication (acute), 80
postpartum psychiatric disorders, 122
pyromania, 57–58
somatic symptom and related disorders, 19
tic disorders, 23
Tourette syndrome, 68
trichotillomania, 128
dying, stages of reaction, 24
dysarthria, as speech disturbance, 78

E

eating, and bulimia nervosa, 231
ECG. *see* electrocardiogram
ECT. *see* electroconvulsive therapy
education
   gender identity disorder, 209
   obsessive-compulsive disorder (OCD), 187
EEG. *see* electroencephalogram
elderly (older than 65). *see also* nursing home patient
   antidepressants, 35–36, 37
   Behavioural Dyscontrol Scale, 158
   cardiovascular changes, 84–85
   Clifton Assessment Procedures for the Elderly, 158
   and cognitive behavioural therapy (CBT), 247
   cognitive functions changes, 129
   cognitive impairment (mild), 81
   dementia, 126
   depression, 126
   executive function, 129
   memory, 129
   motor speed, 129
   neuropsychological tests, 119–120
   psychometric tests, 157–158
   reaction time, 129
   retrograde memory loss, 26–27
   sertraline, 37
   sleep changes, 71
electric shock therapy, for depression and mania, 226
electrocardiogram (ECG), and arrhythmia, 243
electroconvulsive therapy (ECT)
   characteristics as treatment, 60
   cognitive effects, 60
   complications, 14
   features, 101–102
   indications and contraindications, 58
   information to cover, 227
   and lithium, 60
   neurotransmitter changes, 143
   observation of patient, 227
   and schizophrenia, 58, 101–102
   side effects, 227
   and treatment-resistant depression (TRD), 226
electroencephalogram (EEG)
   and lithium, 116
   and neurotransmitters, 106
   waves in, 61–62
emergency, reaction to, 201
endocrine system, effect of lithium, 116
enuresis
   characteristics, 152–153
   etiologic and risk factors, 172–173
   primary *vs.* secondary, 172
epidemiological data, mood disorders, 151–152
epidemiological studies, observed associations, 157
epigenetic model of development, stages, 103–104
Erikson, Erik, 69, 103–104
Erikson's epigenetic model of development, stages of, 103–104
escitalopram, withdrawal symptoms, 30
executive function
   changes in elderly, 129
   tests, 120
externalizing behaviours, rating scales, 66

F

factitious disorder, in *DSM-5*, 19
family and family support
   alcohol dependence of patient, 190–191

and anorexia nervosa, 82
and bulimia nervosa, 231
characteristics of alcoholism, 72
domestic violence, 191
education during treatment, 187, 190
gender identity disorder, 209
history of mental illness and attachment problems, 181–183
family structure and family structure therapy, 129–130, 174
fathers, of children with conduct disorder, 68
fitness to stand trial, McCarty criteria, 178
5-HT (5-HIAA), in etiology of depression, 170
5-HT receptors, and electroconvulsive therapy (ECT), 143
fluctuating cognitive impairment, in normal pressure hydrocephalus (NPH), 27
fluoxetine
  and carbamazepine, 43
  plasma levels of methadone, 103
  withdrawal symptoms, 30
fluvoxamine, and carbamazepine, 43
folie à deux, features, 166
folie simultanée, features, 166
food, tyramine in, 161
foster family, biopsychosocial factors, 221–222
fragile X syndrome (FXS)
  description and features, 109
  pairing, 66
Freud, Sigmund, 105, 155
Freudian psychoanalysis, techniques, 113–114
frigophobia, as culture-bound disorder, 78
frontal lobe function, tests, 20, 69–70
frontal lobe syndrome, presentations, 18
frontotemporal lobar degeneration (FTD), diagnostic features, 63–64
FTD. *see* frontotemporal lobar degeneration
FXS. *see* fragile X syndrome

G

GABA. *see* γ-aminobutyric acid
$GABA_A$, and benzodiazepines (BZDs), 15–16, 74
$GABA_B$ and $GABA_C$, and benzodiazepines (BZDs), 15–16
gabapentin, mechanisms and features, 77
galantamine
  for Alzheimer disease, 121
  as cholinesterase inhibitor, 71
  use and side effects, 121
γ-aminobutyric acid (GABA) benzodiazepines (BZDs), 15–16
  and gabapentin, 77
γ-aminobutyric acid (GABA) benzodiazepine receptor complex, and buspirone hydrochloride, 14
Ganser syndrome, features, 120
gender identity disorder/gender dysphoria
  comorbidities, 208
  family involvement and advice to, 209
  patient assessment, 208
  sources of information, 209
General Health Questionnaire (GHQ), for psychiatric rating, 63
genetic traits, conduct disorder, 22
Gerstmann syndrome
  features, 106
  and posterior parietal lobe, 18
GHQ. *see* General Health Questionnaire
Glasgow coma scale, head injuries, 150
glutamate
  and acamprosate, 57
  and memantine, 121
  and obsessive-compulsive disorder (OCD), 38
Go-No-Go task, and frontal lobe function, 70
grief, normal *vs.* prolonged, 194

H

HAD. *see* HIV-associated dementia
hallucinations, and schizophrenia, 124
haloperidol, for Tourette syndrome, 68
HAM-A. *see* Hamilton Anxiety Rating Scale
HAM-D. *see* Hamilton Depression Rating Scale
Hamilton Anxiety Rating Scale (HAM-A), and anxiety disorder, 247
Hamilton Depression Rating Scale (HAM-D), characteristics, 107
Hamilton Depression Rating Scale (HDRS), 66
HDRS. *see* Hamilton Depression Rating Scale
head injuries, psychiatric morbidity, 150
hematological side effects, of carbamazepine, 34–35
hepatic disorders, and acamprosate, 57

hepatotoxicity, drug-induced: risk factors and causes, 104–105
hippocampal lesions, and amnesia, 40–41
histamine H_1, effects of receptor occupancy, 163
HIV-associated dementia (HAD), features, 108
hoarding disorder, description, 159
hormonal changes, in aging, 118
Huntington disease, features and CAGs, 108–109
hyperactivity
 and clonidine, 171
 symptoms, 226
hyperphagia, in Prader-Willi syndrome, 20–21
hypertriglyceridemia, hormonal changes in aging, 118
hypokalemia, and anorexia nervosa, 128–129
hypomania
 and bipolar disorder in children, 21–22
 and lithium, 101
hypothalamic-diencephalic lesions, amnesia, 40–41

I
illness anxiety disorder, in *DSM-5*, 19
impulse-control disorders, kleptomania, 125–126
infants
 alcoholism in mother, 181–183
 separation/individualism theory, 59
informed consent, from patient, 194, 214–215
inositol, for treatment-resistant depression (TRD), 40
insecure attachment, factors, 182
insulin, hormonal changes in aging, 118
intellectual disability
 diagnostic criteria, 150–151
 and Down syndrome, 151
 features, 29
interpersonal psychotherapy (IPT)
 and bulimia nervosa, 231
 as method and treatment, 154–155
intimate partner violence, factors, 191
intractable epilepsy, and electroconvulsive therapy (ECT), 58
intrusive thoughts, differential diagnosis, 186
IPT. *see* interpersonal psychotherapy

irreversible monoamine oxidase inhibitors (irreversible MAOIs), food products to be avoided, 161

K
Klein, Melanie, 69
kleptomania, features, 125–126
Klerman, Gerald, 154
Klüver-Bucy syndrome, features, 147
koro, as culture-bound disorder, 77
Kübler-Ross, Elizabeth, 24

L
L-triiodothyronine (T_3), for treatment-resistant depression (TRD), 40
lamotrigine
 characteristics and side effects, 163
 teratogenicity, 146
language, tests, 174
latah
 conditions and description of, 123
 as culture-bound disorder, 77
life events, and psychiatric disorders, 82–83
lifestyle behaviour, complications, 243
lithium
 brain-derived neurotrophic factor (BDNF), 162
 effects on cardiovascular and endocrine systems, 116
 for electroconvulsive therapy (ECT), 60
 and electroencephalogram (EEG), 116
 intoxication levels and symptoms, 165–166
 number needed to treat (NNT) value, 100–101
 risks and alternative treatments, 194
 teratogenicity, 146
 for treatment-resistant depression (TRD), 40
lithium therapy, mania and manic symptoms, 100–101
lobar atrophy, in Pick disease, 114
logoclonia, as speech disturbance, 78
Luria test, and frontal lobe function, 70

M
MADRS. *see* Montgomery-Asberg Depression Rating Scale
magnetic resonance imaging (MRI), fluctuating cognitive impairment, 27
Mahler, Margaret, 59

major depressive disorder (MDD)
  and body dysmorphic disorder (BDD), 169
  interpersonal psychotherapy (IPT), 155
mania and manic symptoms
  brain-derived neurotrophic factor (BDNF), 162
  and electroconvulsive therapy (ECT), 58
  lithium therapy, 100–101
MAO_A and MAO_B, 15
MAOIs. *see* monoamine oxidase inhibitors
mature defence mechanisms, features, 24–25
McCarty criteria, fitness to stand trial, 178
MCI. *see* mild cognitive impairment
MDD. *see* major depressive disorder
medical conditions, and psychological factors, 18–19
medical emergency, reaction to, 201
medications, course of action, 202
melancholic depression
  signs, 127
  suicide risk, 60–61
  symptoms, 78–79
memantine
  as cholinesterase inhibitor, 71
  features, 120–121
  for obsessive-compulsive disorder (OCD), 38
memory
  assessment tests, 171
  changes in elderly, 129
  neuropsychological tests, 119–120
  test, 174
memory loss, retrograde: symptoms in elderly, 26–27
metacognitive therapy, attention deficit hyperactivity disorder (ADHD), 239–240
methadone
  vs. buprenorphine, 99
  features, 142–143
  as opiate antagonist, 16
  overdose mortality, 142–143
  plasma levels, 103
methylphenidate, for children with ADHD/PATS, 72–73
Michigan Alcohol Screening Test (MAST), 205
mild cognitive impairment (MCI), tests for memory, 171

monoamine oxidase inhibitors, irreversible (irreversible MAOIs), food products to be avoided, 161
monoamine oxidase inhibitors (MAOIs)
  characteristics, 15
  combination therapy limitations, 31
  side effects and characteristics, 31
Montgomery-Asberg Depression Rating Scale (MADRS), features, 148
mood disorders, epidemiological data, 151–152
mood stabilizers
  features, 75
  teratogenicity, 146
mothers
  of children with conduct disorder, 68
  and psychosis, 217–218
motor speed, changes in elderly, 129
motor tic disorders, characteristics, 22–23
MRI. *see* magnetic resonance imaging
muscarinic M_1, effects of receptor occupancy, 163

N
N-acetylaspartate
  and electroconvulsive therapy (ECT), 143
  for obsessive-compulsive disorder (OCD), 38
naloxone, as opiate antagonist, 16
naltrexone
  as opiate antagonist, 16
  relapse of alcoholism, 206
  side effects, 16
narcolepsy, psychostimulants, 24
negative automatic thoughts, 114
neglect
  biopsychosocial aspects, 221–222
  impact in adulthood, 223
  psychodynamic factors, 223
neuroleptic-induced tardive dyskinesia: mechanisms, risks, and symptoms, 153–154
neuroleptic malignant syndrome (NMS)
  and electroconvulsive therapy (ECT), 58
  management principles, 201
  symptoms, 83–84
neuroleptic withdrawal-emergent dyskinesia, features, 154
neuroleptics, for obsessive-compulsive disorder (OCD), 85

neuropsychological tests, for memory, 119–120
neurotransmitters
  and electroconvulsive therapy (ECT), 143
  and electroencephalograms (EEG), 106
nightmares, characteristics, 39
NIMH. *see* US National Institute of Mental Health
NMS. *see* neuroleptic malignant syndrome
NNT. *see* number needed to treat
normal grief, characteristics, 194
normal pressure hydrocephalus (NPH)
  characteristics, 27
  features and symptoms, 65
normal sleep, features, 17–18
NPH. *see* normal pressure hydrocephalus
number needed to treat (NNT) value
  for antidepressants, 72
  lithium, 100–101
nursing home patient, disruptive behaviours
  detailed management, 213–214
  differential diagnoses, 213
  investigations, 213

O

obsession and compulsion, causes, 41–42
obsessive-compulsive disorder (OCD)
  and body dysmorphic disorder (BDD), 122, 169
  brain regions involved, 76–77
  as chronic condition, 99–100
  family education and support, 187
  features, 100
  and glutamate, 38
  hoarding disorder, 159
  management of presentation, 186–187
  neuroleptics, 85
  Pediatric OCD Treatment Study (POTS), 73–74
  prognostic factors, 156
  and selective serotonin reuptake inhibitors (SSRIs), 85
  sexual thoughts, 186
  and stalking, 169
  suicide risk, 61
  treatments, 38, 186–187
  trichotillomania, 128
obsessive-compulsive personality disorder (OCPD)
  and body dysmorphic disorder (BDD), 82
  as chronic condition, 99–100
  features, 100, 113
OCD. *see* obsessive-compulsive disorder
OCPD. *see* obsessive-compulsive personality disorder
Oedipus conflict, resolution, 83
opiate intoxication, symptoms, 142
opiate withdrawal, symptoms, 142
opioid-addiction treatment, and opioid antagonists, 16
opioid intoxication, indicators, 25
opioid overdose, signs, 80, 159
opioid withdrawal, buprenorphine and methadone, 99
overdose, assessment, 230
overweight, complications, 243

P

P value, in statistical terminology, 19–20
PANDAS. *see* pediatric autoimmune neuropsychiatric disorders associated with streptococcal infections
panic disorder
  suicidal ideation factors, 33
  suicide risk, 61
paranoid personality disorder, features, 113
paraphasic errors, Wernicke dysphasia, 173
parents, of children with conduct disorder, 68
parietal lobe lesions, presentations, 18
patients
  competence in decision making and participation, 124–125, 200
  informed consent, 194, 214–215
  observation by medical students, 227
  questions about suicidal ideation factors, 193
  transference feelings, 205
PATS. *see* Preschool ADHD Treatment Study
PCP. *see* phencyclidine (PCP) intoxication
PDD. *see* persistent depressive disorder
Pearson product moment correlation, 149
pediatric autoimmune neuropsychiatric disorders associated with streptococcal infections (PANDAS), clinical characteristics, 111–112
Pediatric OCD Treatment Study (POTS), conclusions, 73–74
perception tests, descriptions, 173–174
persistent depressive disorder (PDD), features, 110–111

persistent motor disorder, characteristics, 23
personality disorders, pairs and
  features, 113
pharmacokinetics, physiologic
  characteristics, 160–161
phencyclidine (PCP) intoxication, signs,
  80, 159
phenobarbital, plasma levels of
  methadone, 103
phenytoin, plasma levels of methadone, 103
PHQ-9 score, 193
Pick disease
  features, 148–149
  and lobar atrophy, 114
pindolol, for treatment-resistant
  depression (TRD) and SSRIs, 40
postpartum depression, history of, 217
postpartum psychiatric disorders, risks
  and presentations, 122
postpartum psychosis, incidence and
  presentations, 122
posttraumatic stress disorder (PTSD)
  risk factors, 117
  suicide risk, 61
  symptoms, 84
  trauma-focused cognitive behavioural
    therapy (TF-CBT), 37–38
POTS. see Pediatric OCD Treatment Study
power of hypothesis, in statistical
  terminology, 19–20
Prader-Willi syndrome
  clinical features, 20–21
  pairing, 66
pregnancy
  and alcoholism, 181
  and psychosis, 217–218
  and psychosis relapse, 218
  substance use tools, 205
Preschool ADHD Treatment Study
  (PATS), findings, 72–73
Present State Examination (PSE), for
  psychiatric rating, 63
primary enuresis, 172
primary motor dysphasia (Broca
  dysphasia), findings, 173
prolonged grief disorder, characteristics, 194
propranolol, for antipsychotic-induced
  akathisia, 164
PSE. see Present State Examination
psychiatric disorders
  and life events, 82–83
  suicide risk, 60–61
psychiatric morbidity, head injuries, 150

psychiatric rating, scales of measurement,
  62–63
psychiatric unit, transfer of patients, 201
psychoanalysis, techniques, 113–114
psychological factors, and medical
  conditions, 18–19
psychometric tests, cognitive functions,
  157–158
psychosexual evaluation, elements, 208
psychosis
  after birth, 217–218
  and arrhythmia, 243
  differential diagnosis, 184
  follow-up care, 243–244
  medication and breastfeeding, 217–218
  pharmacological management, 217
  post-medication management, 218
  prodromal symptoms, 36
  relapses, 218
  safety of patient and baby, 217
  tests and antibiotics, 243
  and trichotillomania, 128
psychosocial development model, phases
  and age range, 105
psychostimulants, side effects, 23–24
psychotherapy, for bulimia nervosa, 231
psychotic disorders
  characteristics, 75–76
  progression to full-blown disorders, 172
  substance-induced vs. non-substance-
    induced, 197
psychotropic medications
  and breastfeeding, 217–218
  disruptive behaviour disorder, 30
PTSD. see posttraumatic stress disorder
pyromania, definition and characteristics,
  57–58

Q
quetiapine, for Tourette syndrome, 68

R
rapid cycling, definition and risk factors, 13
rash, and lamotrigine, 163
reaction time, changes in elderly, 129
reality distortion symptoms,
  schizophrenia, 124
receptor occupancy, and antipsychotics,
  162–163
refeeding syndrome: features, monitoring,
  and prevention, 233
relapse prevention, alcoholism and alcohol
  dependence, 205

reproducing interlocking pentagons, and visuospatial skills, 69
retrograde memory loss, symptoms in elderly, 26–27
riluzole, for obsessive-compulsive disorder (OCD), 38
risperidone
   disruptive behaviour disorder, 30
   plasma levels of methadone, 103
   for Tourette syndrome, 68
rivastigmine, as cholinesterase inhibitor, 71
Rogers, Carl, 69

S
schizoaffective disorder
   antipsychotics, 201–202
   blood report, 200–201
   differential diagnoses, 200
   investigations, 200
   management, 201
schizoid personality disorder, features, 113
schizophrenia
   and clozapine, 250–251, 252
   differential diagnoses, 197
   and electroconvulsive therapy (ECT), 58, 101–102
   first-rank symptoms, 32
   predictive factors, 172
   prognostic factors, 144–145
   reality distortion symptoms, 124
   and speech disturbances, 78
   substance use, 197
   suicide risk factors, 167–168
schizophrenia, chronic: indicators, 126–127
schizotypal personality disorder, features, 113
Schneiderian criteria, schizophrenia, 32
Schwann cells, 107
secondary enuresis, 172
secure attachment, compromising factors, 221–222
security, against violent patients, 177–178, 198
seizures, and clozapine, 116
selective serotonin reuptake inhibitors (SSRIs)
   neuroleptics, 85
   number needed to treat (NNT) value, 72
   for obsessive-compulsive disorder (OCD), 85, 187
   pindolol, 40

sexual side effects, 80
side effects, 80, 144
withdrawal symptoms, 29–30
sensitivity, definition and description, 123, 149
separation/individualism theory, process, 59
serotonin 5-HT, effects of receptor occupancy, 162–163
serotonin-norepinephrine reuptake inhibitors (SNRIs)
   number needed to treat (NNT) value, 72
   sexual side effects, 80
sertraline
   for elderly, 37
   for obsessive-compulsive disorder (OCD), 73–74
   plasma levels of methadone, 103
sexual abuse, impact in adulthood, 223
sexual identity, differential diagnoses, 208
sexual offences, intrusive thoughts, 186
sinus node dysfunction, and lithium, 116
65+. *see* elderly (older than 65)
sleep
   changes in elderly, 71
   features, 17–18
   spindles, 147
   stages, 147
sleep electroencephalogram (EEG), and neurotransmitters, 106
sleep terrors, characteristics, 39
SNRIs. *see* serotonin-norepinephrine reuptake inhibitors
social anxiety disorder, and body dysmorphic disorder (BDD), 169
Social Readjustment Rating Scale, for stressful life changes, 82–83
somatic symptom disorder, in *DSM-5*, 19
Spearman rank correlation, description, 149
specificity, definition and description, 124, 149
speech disturbances, and schizophrenia, 78
SSRIs. *see* selective serotonin reuptake inhibitors
STAI. *see* State-Trait Anxiety Inventory
stalking, estimates and features, 169–170
State-Trait Anxiety Inventory (STAI), 247
statistical concepts, descriptions, 149
statistical terminology, descriptions in, 19–20
stimulants, cardiac effects, 74–75

Stroop Color-Word Test, for frontal lobe function, 171
structural family therapy, elements, 129–130, 174
stuttering, as speech disturbance, 78
subcortical dementia, features, 65
sublimation
 as defence mechanism, 155
 against stressors, 155
substance use
 consequences of using multiple substances, 197–198
 differential diagnoses, 197
 history of and questions to patient, 204
 and psychotic disorders, 197
 and schizophrenia, 197
 screening tools, 204–205
substance-use disorders, and body dysmorphic disorder (BDD), 169
suicidal ideation factors
 and body dysmorphic disorder (BDD), 169
 in panic disorder, 33
 questions to patient, 193
suicide
 assessment of attempted suicide, 230
 biopsychosocial aspects, 221–222
 and body dysmorphic disorder (BDD), 169
 differential diagnoses, 231
 and lithium therapy, 101
 psychiatric disorders and depression, 60–61
 risk factors in schizophrenia, 167–168
syndromes, chromosomal abnormality in, 66–67

T
T_3. see L-triiodothyronine
T_4. see thyroxine
tacrine, for Alzheimer disease/use and side effects, 121
tardive dyskinesia (TD), symptoms and characteristics, 164–165
TD. see tardive dyskinesia
temperamental variables, 17
teratogenicity, in mood stabilizers, 146
TF-CBT. see trauma-focused cognitive behavioural therapy
theory-author pairings, 69
thiamine, and Wernicke encephalopathy, 35
Thomas, Alexander, 17
3A4, and carbamazepine, 75
thyroid gland, changes in aging, 127
thyroid hormone augmentation, for treatment-resistant depression (TRD), 40
thyroxine (T_4), for treatment-resistant depression (TRD), 40
tic disorders, characteristics, 22–23
Token Test, 174
Tourette disorder, and basal ganglia, 23
Tourette syndrome
 symptoms, 68–69
 treatment, 68
Trail Making Test, Part B, in frontal lobe functioning, 20
transference feelings, 205
trauma-focused cognitive behavioural therapy (TF-CBT), components, 37–38
TRD. see treatment-resistant depression
treatment-resistant depression (TRD)
 augmentation strategies and agents, 39–40
 and electroconvulsive therapy (ECT), 226
 management steps, 31
 psychostimulants, 24
 treatment failure reasons, 30–31
 treatment options, 226
 warning signs, 226
treatments
 competency of patient, 200
 informed consent, 194
trichotillomania, features, 128
TWEAK (drug-abuse screening test), 205
type I and type II alcoholism, features, 168
type I and type II errors, in statistical terminology, 19–20
tyramine, in foods, 161

U
uncomplicated grief, characteristics, 194
unipolar depression, lithium therapy, 100–101
US National Institute of Mental Health (NIMH), PATS, 72–73

V
valproic acid, teratogenicity, 146
valproate, brain-derived neurotrophic factor (BDNF), 162

vascular dementia, neuroimaging findings, 70
violence
    alcoholism and alcohol dependence, 205
    differential diagnoses, 177
    domestic, 191
    patient management and treatment, 177–178, 198
    persistence, 81
    protective factors, 81
    response to, 198
    and staff safety, 177–178
Visual Object and Space Perception Battery, as test, 174
visuospatial skills, tasks, 69
vocal tic disorder, characteristics, 23
vocal tics, and Tourette syndrome, 68

W

WBC. *see* white blood cell count
WCST. *see* Wisconsin Card-Sorting Test
Weissman, Myrna, 154
Wender Utah Rating Scale, for ADHD, 239
Wernicke dysphasia, findings and paraphasic errors, 173
Wernicke encephalopathy, changes and signs, 35
white blood cell count (WBC), and clozapine, 252
Wilson disease, characteristics, 27
windigo, as culture-bound disorder, 77
Winnicot, Donald, 69
Wisconsin Card-Sorting Test (WCST), in frontal lobe functioning, 20

Y

Y-BOCS. *see* Yale-Brown Obsessive Compulsive Scale
Yale-Brown Obsessive Compulsive Scale (Y-BOCS), and riluzole, 38
Yalom's curative factors, 31–32
young. *see* adolescents; children
Youth Self-Report (YSR), 66